# Clean Needle Technique Manual for Acupuncturists

......................................................

*Guidelines and Standards*
*for the Clean and Safe*
*Clinical Practice of Acupuncture*

......................................................

**FIFTH EDITION**

National Acupuncture Foundation

The clean needle technique protocols set forth in this manual are intended as a general, informative guide for professional colleagues. They are not intended to be enacted into law.

**NAF Publications**
© 2003, 2005 National Acupuncture Foundation
All rights reserved.
Printed in the United States of America
08 07 06 05    2 3 4 5 6

ISBN 0-9670262-6-1

**Acknowledgments**

The five editions of this manual represent the collective thinking and energy of National Acupuncture Foundation Board Members, NCCAOM Commissioners, Council of Colleges of Acupuncture and Oriental Medicine Clean Needle Technique Committee Members and Instructors, and colleagues across the United States. The National Acupuncture Foundation Board Members involved include Malvin Finkelstein, L.Ac; Barbara Mitchell, J.D., L.Ac., (Editor, fourth and fifth edition); William Skelton, L.Ac. and James Turner, J.D. The roll call of the Commissioners of the National Certification Commission for Acupuncture and Oriental Medicine (NCCAOM) involved in the process includes June Brazil, L.Ac.; Edith Davis (Editor); Glenn Earl,Ac.; Steven Finando, Ph.D., L.Ac.; Alan Francis; Daniel Jiao, L.Ac.; Stuart Kutchins, L.Ac.; Jim McCormick, L.Ac. (Editor); Mark Seem, Ph.D., L.Ac.; Angela Tu, L.Ac. and Grace Wong, L.Ac.

Other professionals who made valuable contributions include Ann Bailey, L.Ac.; Matthew Bauer, L.Ac.; Jenny Belluomini,N.D.; Ralph Coan,M.D.; Gary Dolowitz, M.D.; Robert Duggan, L.Ac.; Kevin Ergil, L.Ac.; Steve Given, L.Ac.; Martha Howard,M.D. (Editor); Haig Ignatius,M.D.; Joseph Kay, L.Ac.; Deke Kendall, L.Ac.; Patricia Klucas, R.N.; Su Liang Ku, C.A.; Shen Ping Liang, L.Ac.; William Mueller, L.Ac.; Tom Riihimaki; Ron Sokolsky; Tierney Tully, M.S.O.M.; Brooke Winter, L.Ac.; Julie Zinkus, L.Ac., and Walter Bond of the Centers for Disease Control.

Manual design by Gary Niemeier

# Table of Contents

PREFACE TO THE FIFTH EDITION . . . . . . . . . . . . . . . . . . . . . . . . . . . . . . . . . . . . . . . . . . . . . . . . . . . . . . . . . . . . . . . . v

INTRODUCTION . . . . . . . . . . . . . . . . . . . . . . . . . . . . . . . . . . . . . . . . . . . . . . . . . . . . . . . . . . . . . . . . . . . . . . . . . . . . vii

CHAPTER ONE: The Need for Clean Needle Technique . . . . . . . . . . . . . . . . . . . . . . . . . . . . . . . . . . . . 1

CHAPTER TWO: CNT Protocols . . . . . . . . . . . . . . . . . . . . . . . . . . . . . . . . . . . . . . . . . . . . . . . . . . . . . . . . 13

CHAPTER THREE: Applying CNT in an Acupuncture Treatment . . . . . . . . . . . . . . . . . . . . . . . . . 20

CHAPTER FOUR: Protocols for Sterilizing Instruments . . . . . . . . . . . . . . . . . . . . . . . . . . . . . . . . . 37

CHAPTER FIVE: Risk Reduction . . . . . . . . . . . . . . . . . . . . . . . . . . . . . . . . . . . . . . . . . . . . . . . . . . . . . . . 47

CHAPTER SIX: What to do for: Accidents, etc. . . . . . . . . . . . . . . . . . . . . . . . . . . . . . . . . . . . . . . . . . . 53

CHAPTER SEVEN: Safety Issues when Using Special Techniques . . . . . . . . . . . . . . . . . . . . . . . . . 58

APPENDIX 1: Where to Find More Information . . . . . . . . . . . . . . . . . . . . . . . . . . . . . . . . . . . . . . . . . 60

BIBLIOGRAPHY . . . . . . . . . . . . . . . . . . . . . . . . . . . . . . . . . . . . . . . . . . . . . . . . . . . . . . . . . . . . . . . . . . . . . 61

INDEX . . . . . . . . . . . . . . . . . . . . . . . . . . . . . . . . . . . . . . . . . . . . . . . . . . . . . . . . . . . . . . . . . . . . . . . . . . . . . . 63

# Preface to the Fifth Edition

THE INITIAL CONCEPT OF A manual for clean needle technique evolved out of the landmark development of standards for safe and competent acupuncture practice developed by the National Certification Commission for Acupuncture and Oriental Medicine (NCCAOM) in 1984. These standards were reflected in the first national examination for certification of acupuncturists in the United States in 1985. The knowledge and skills necessary for safe and competent acupuncture practice were identified through a series of surveys and conferences involving experienced practitioners throughout the United States. It was recognized that a variety of styles have evolved in different countries over the centuries, and that all of these have had their influence on acupuncture practice in the United States today. In the development of national standards for the practice of acupuncture, a great effort was made to reflect this diversity.

Standards for clean needle technique are another story. Here the NCCAOM and, subsequently, the National Acupuncture Foundation (NAF) have a responsibility to reflect not the variety of ancient traditions, but rather the most up-to-date information Western science has to offer. Consequently, in this publication, footnotes refer to sources such as the Centers for Disease Control and Prevention (CDCP) and Occupational Safety and Health Administration (OSHA), not to sources such as the *Nei Jing*.

In a society that is presently very concerned about the dangers of communicable diseases, the NAF has taken responsibility for sorting out clinical behaviors in order to identify a safe, practical approach that will protect the public health without burdening practitioners with procedures that go beyond the necessary precautions. In this manual traditional practices are described in the light of practice standards in the acupuncture community and ways are suggested to achieve the greatest practical risk reduction of disease transmission during acupuncture treatment. The recommendations and guidelines contained in this manual have been the basis for a nationally accepted protocol for the safe practice of acupuncture since 1985 and have been instrumental in maintaining an appropriate standard of care.

In the preparation of this fifth edition, the NAF has drawn on a body of clinical and regulatory information regarding communicable diseases that has changed dramatically in the last five years. Readers should continue to keep themselves current on the latest developments in regulation as well as infection control and reflect these developments in their practice.

This edition has been substantially reorganized to integrate OSHA codes and the latest information on communicable diseases.

This manual is intended to be used as a reference by every acupuncturist because it includes new information that is important to experienced as well as new practitioners. The intent is not to dictate a single style of clinical procedure, but rather to provide information about sterility, asepsis, hygienic practices and practical clinical guidelines that can serve as the basis for intelligent individual judgment.

The information included in the manual is also of importance to acupuncturists' assistants and office staff. Anyone who works in a health care office must understand the concepts of communicable diseases and medical waste management and their place in ensuring maximum reduction of risk of cross-infection for both staff and patients.

The NAF has drawn on a wide range of source materials in the preparation of this manual. The NAF has made every effort to retain only those recommendations that experts consider important for the protection of the patient and the practitioner. Reasons are given for each recommendation. All acupuncture practitioners are urged to take them seriously and make a strong commitment to change procedures when necessary. Adherence to clean needle technique ensures both public and practitioner safety and is in the best interest of the public, the practitioner, and the acupuncture profession.

Barbara B. Mitchell, J.D., L.Ac.
Editor

# Introduction

IN 1984, AT THE REQUEST OF THE acupuncture profession, the National Certification Commission for Acupuncture and Oriental Medicine addressed the issue of clean needle technique and developed guidelines and recommendations for the safe and clean practice of acupuncture. The guidelines are based on sound scientific evidence where possible or on solid theory supported by the opinion of experts in the field of public health. Conscientious use of the procedures recommended and described in this manual will reduce the risk of spreading infection and the risk of accidents within the acupuncture setting. The National Acupuncture Foundation (NAF) has continued to revise and update the *Clean Needle Technique Manual* to reflect the changes in knowledge and practice.

Every increase in the knowledge and application of safe clinical practices and risk management techniques reduces the risk of spread of infection and helps ensure public safety. Furthermore, from the medical, legal and ethical perspectives, it is the practitioner's responsibility to demonstrate that proper sterilization and clean needle technique have been followed correctly.

In developing these protocols, the NAF has drawn from techniques developed and scientifically tested by experts in infection control. These include the Centers for Disease Control and Prevention in Atlanta, Georgia, the Occupational Safety and Health Administration's Bloodborne Pathogens Standards and the U.S. Public Health Service. The NAF welcomes their expertise, has adapted to the practice of acupuncture many of the techniques suggested for other professions, and thanks these agencies for their work and support. Thus, many of the recommendations in this manual are modified versions of techniques currently in use throughout the United States in other health care professions. In addition, Oriental works on the subject and the clinical experience of professional acupuncturists have been used to develop this manual. The guidelines and standards that have been developed thus combine Oriental and Western resources.

CHAPTER **1**

# The Need for Clean Needle Technique

It is essential that practitioners understand the mechanisms of disease transmission and know the characteristics of infectious diseases, particularly hepatitis and HIV, which are of particular concern in the health care setting. This knowledge underscores the need to use clean needle technique procedures for the protection of patients, practitioners and staff.

## THE IMMUNE RESPONSE TO PATHOGENS

From a clean needle technique perspective, the primary purpose of the body's immune system is to respond to the introduction of pathogenic organisms.

The body is constantly exposed to infectious agents, some of which are normally found in or on specific areas of the body, especially on the skin, in the mouth, respiratory passageways, urinary tract, colon and mucous membranes of the eyes. Many of these organisms that are normally present are capable of causing disease if they invade other tissues or if the immune system is ineffective in controlling the infectious agent. In addition, a person is intermittently exposed to virulent bacteria and viruses from outside the body that can cause specific diseases, such as pneumonia, streptococcal and staphylococcal infections, and typhoid fever. These infectious agents may be very invasive and overcome the natural barriers to infection.

Natural barriers include intact skin and mucous membranes of the nose, throat, urethra, and rectum. They include stomach acid, which kills many swallowed microbes by lowering gastric pH. They include healthy cells of the nose and lungs, which can expel inhaled pathogens. They include normal mucus and saliva, which can coat and neutralize many germs. Nonspecific factors in the immune response that protect the body from invasion and infection are the activity of the epithelial skin layer and mucus membranes, and the cleansing effects of tears, urine, and acidity of vaginal secretions.

Microbes can enter the body through a break in the skin, such as a cut or wound, or through the orifices (mouth, nose, urethra, etc.). Any infectious agents, including bacterial spores, can cause infection if they contact areas of the body that are not their natural habitat.

There are many potential sources of infectious disease in an acupuncture office. These include hands, blood, saliva, nasal and other bodily secretions, dust, clothing and hair. Infections associated with acupuncture practice may be classified into two types according to the source of the disease agent — autogenous and cross-infections.

## Autogenous Infections

These are infections caused by pathogens that the patient is already carrying. An example of this would be peritonitis following a deep abdominal insertion that punctures the peritoneum and the intestine. The bacteria that are normal to the intestinal tract are then able to invade the peritoneal cavity, resulting in infection. The incidence of autogenous infection from acupuncture may be low, but the consequences can be catastrophic.

One of the dangers of reusing a needle during treatment is that infectious agents natural to one location can be transferred to another that does not have the same natural flora or defenses and is thus vulnerable to infection.

## Cross-Infections

These infections are caused by pathogens acquired from another person or by the environment. They may be acquired directly (e.g. from contact between patient and practitioner), or by transfer (e.g. carried from one patient to another on the unwashed hands of the practitioner). Cross-infections may be acquired by the practitioner and office personnel as well as by patients. Two of the most serious are hepatitis B virus and HIV. Tuberculosis is also becoming a growing public health concern in the United States.

Under normal circumstances natural barriers prevent the infectious agent or virus from causing an infection. But when the natural defenses are weakened, or the infectious agent is of a density, or bioload, great enough to overwhelm the body's defenses, the invasion can result in disease. As a practitioner, the acupuncturist must always be alert to the potential for transferring disease-causing agents to patients.

An infectious agent can travel from one host to another in a variety of ways, including being carried on dust or droplets of moisture in the air, being transferred in body fluids, and by mechanical transfer from one surface to another. The density of a infectious agent is one of the factors in risk of cross-infection. Where one cell of a disease-causing agent might be easily coped with in a healthy body, a droplet that is teeming with infectious agents could be more than the body can handle. For example, the hepatitis virus is a high-density virus, which explains why it is one of the most easily transferred diseases.

# HEPATITIS

There are several subtypes of the hepatitis virus: A, B, C, D, and E. Hepatitis A and E are transmitted mainly via fecal-contaminated food and water. The others are transmitted by blood and/or sexual exposure. Hepatitis is such a concern in a health care setting that the Occupational Safety and Health Administration (OSHA) has adopted specific language regarding the transmission of hepatitis and recommendations for training and vaccination of staff. The Center for Disease Control and Prevention (CDCP) strongly recommends that all health care workers be vaccinated for hepatitis B. CDCP states that the highest risks occur during the professional training period; therefore, vaccination should be completed while in school.[1]

## Hepatitis A (HAV)

Hepatitis A (HAV, formerly called infectious hepatitis or short-incubation hepatitis) is a common infection in conditions of poor sanitation and overcrowding. Although transmission is mainly via fecal-contaminated food and water, virus in the bloodstream and on hands poses a potential hazard in acupuncture practice. Good personal hygiene and proper sanitation can help prevent hepatitis A.

The incubation period of HAV is 15 to 50 days, with an average incubation period of 28 days.[2] Unlike hepatitis B (HBV) or C (HCV), onset is abrupt. Other symptoms include abdominal discomfort, loss of appetite, fatigue, nausea, dark urine and jaundice. Symptoms usually last less than 2 months. Although there is no chronic infection, approximately 15% of people infected have a prolonged or relapsing course of illness lasting as long as 6-9 months. Individuals who have had HAV cannot be reinfected.

HAV is most frequently found in children and young adults with the number of cases tending to peak during the autumn. The CDCP says that 23,000 cases are officially reported each year, but estimates that one-third of Americans have evidence of past infection (immunity).[3] Fortunately most cases are relatively mild, complications are uncommon, and chronic carrier states are not known.

There is now a vaccination for HAV[4] but CDCP does not routinely recommend HAV vaccination for health care workers since they are not at increased risk.[5] Routine infection control precautions will prevent transmission.

---

1. Centers for Disease Control and Prevention, Immunization of Health-Care Workers: Recommendations of the Advisory Committee on Immunization Practices (ACIP) and the Hospital Infection Control Practices Advisory Committee (HICPAC), MMR 1997; 46 (No. RR18).

2. See http://www.cdc.gov/ncidod/diseases/hepatitis/a/faqa.htm for information on HAV for practitioners and consumers

3. http://www.cdc.gov/ncidod/diseases/hepatitis/a/fact.htm

4. "On May 11, 2001, the FDA licensed a combined hepatitis A and B Twinrix® vaccine for use in persons aged greater than 18. The antigenic components in Twinrix® have been used routinely in separately single antigen vaccines in the Unites States since 1995 and 1989 as hepatitis A & B vaccines respectively." http://www.cdc.gov/ncid

5. Individuals with increased risk include those working or traveling in a country with high or intermediate rates of HAV, illegal drug users, for men who have sex with men and for individuals with chronic liver disease. See http://www.cdc.gov/ncidod/diseases/hepatitis/a/faqa.htm for further information.

# Hepatitis B (HBV)

Hepatitis B virus (HBV, serum hepatitis or long-incubation hepatitis) is the major bloodborne pathogen presenting a risk of infection in an acupuncture clinic. HBV is the second sub-type of hepatitis for which a vaccine exists. HBV is associated with lifelong infection, cirrhosis (scarring) of the liver, liver cancer, liver failure and death.

> Hepatitis B is the most significant infectious occupational risk in the United States.

## Transmission of HBV

HBV is highly contagious. It is spread through casual contact as well as direct contact with contaminated blood and body fluids. Food and water can become contaminated with HBV where proper sanitation is lacking. Infected individuals should be isolated or follow careful infection prevention procedures, especially during home care. The infected person should not share food or drink with family members and all eating and drinking utensils used by the infected person should be washed in hot soapy water. These precautionary measures should be followed until the person tests negative.

## Individuals at Risk of HBV Infection

In 1999, an estimated 80,000 people in the U.S were infected with HBV. One out of 20 people in the United States will get infected with HBV some time during their lives. Approximately 5,000 people each year die due to HBV.[6]

Individuals most at risk of HBV infection are those who come into frequent contact with blood and blood products, such as health care workers (physicians, dentists, nurses, blood bank workers, paramedical personnel, laboratory staff) or patients and their contacts.[7] The risk of HBV infection in the workplace is primarily related to the degree of contact with blood in the workplace and to the HBV status of the source person.[8]

One of the most common modes of HBV transmission in the health care setting is the unintentional injury of a health care worker from a needle contaminated with HbeAg-positive blood from an infected patient.[9] The CDCP estimates that 8,700 health care workers become infected with HBV each year, that 2,100 will have acute hepatitis, approximately 400 of them will be hospitalized and that approximately 200 will die from effects of acute and chronic HBV infection.[10]

---

6.  http://www.cdc.gov/ncidod/diseases/hepatitis/b/faqb.htm (April 14, 2002)

7.  The incidence of HBV infections among health care workers has decreased substantially from the early 1980's. This is attributed to the implementation of standards precautions, including barrier precautions, and increasing levels of hepatitis B vaccination coverage among HCWs. Beltrami, EM, Williams IT, Shapiro, CN and Chamberland, ME, "Risk and Management of Blood-Borne Infections in Health Care Workers," *Clinical Microbiology Reviews* 13, No. 3 (July 2000).

8.  MMWR 6/29/01 50 (RR11);1-42

9.  Beltrani, *op. cite.*

10. The Bloodborne Pathogens Standard, A Pragmatic Approach, Jon T. O'Neal, M.D., M.P.H., Van Nostrand Reinhold, New York, page 9 (1996)

Other groups at risk include those who live in crowded or unsanitary conditions (including prisoners and certain immigrant populations), have many sexual contacts, are a man and have sex with a man, live in the same house with someone who has chronic HBV, have sex with someone infected with HBV, have hemophilia, are a patient or work in a home for the developmentally disabled, travel to areas where hepatitis B is endemic, are IV drug users or have several of these risk factors.[11]

> To minimize the risk of HBV transmission, health care workers should adhere to universal precautions, including appropriate handwashing, protective barriers and care in the use and disposal of needles.

### Exposure to HBV

Health care workers are at a much higher risk for HBV infection than the general public due to their frequent occupational exposure to blood and blood products as well as other body fluids. Studies in numerous medical journals, such as the *New England Journal of Medicine* and the *Journal of the American Medical Association,* reveal a high rate of HBV infection among health care professionals working in their field.

Hepatitis B must be recognized as an occupational hazard for acupuncturists, as it is for other health care professionals whose procedures commonly include the penetration of the skin or cause exposure to bodily fluids. Invasive procedures, where there is considerable risk of exposure to contaminated blood and body fluids, pose the greatest risk of occupational infection from HBV. CDCP strongly recommends that all personnel working in such areas should scrupulously follow universal precautions. Disposable equipment and protective clothing should be used whenever possible and proper disinfecting and sterilization by autoclaving should be standard policy for nondisposable equipment.

> CDCP recommends that health care workers be vaccinated against HBV, always follow universal precautions and handle needles safely.

### Vaccination

A vaccine against hepatitis B was developed in 1981. One to two months after an individual receives the complete series of three injections, the HBsAb test will reveal if immunity has been achieved. An elevated HBsAb titer indicates immunity.

Vaccination is recommended for personnel performing invasive procedures, cleaning contaminated equipment or performing duties in an area where there is a risk of exposure. CDCP recommends that all health care workers be vaccinated against HBV and OSHA requires all employers to offer HBV vaccination to personnel performing invasive procedures or cleaning contaminated equipment.[12] In October 1997, the Advisory Committee on Immunization Practices expanded its hepatitis B vaccination recommendations to include all children aged 0-18 years.

11. Ibid. footnote 4

12. OSHA also requires that employees receive bloodborne pathogen education prior to having contact with blood or body fluids.

Five years after vaccination the immunity might begin to diminish. Individuals who wish to determine their HBV status should have an antibody titer measured. Those vaccinated for HBV four or five years earlier should have titers measured periodically to determine if a booster course of the vaccine may be needed.

**The HBV Infection Process**

The incubation period for HBV is 50 to 180 days. During this period, the infectious virus appears in the blood and saliva, and it may appear in the feces, urine, semen, tears, and even sweat. During this period the infection may be spread even though no symptoms are present.

> "HBV is easier to catch than HIV because it is over 100 times more concentrated in an infected person's blood and it can exist on surfaces outside the body."
>
> http://www.immunize.org/catg.d/p4115.htm

HBV early symptoms often begin with mild flu-like signs and symptoms such as a fever (in 60% of cases), general malaise, or insidious onset of anorexia and abdominal pain. Other symptoms may include chills, nausea, joint pains, rash, and diarrhea. Typically these symptoms last from two to six weeks. These symptoms are frequently followed by a period of extreme fatigue and depression that can extend for several months.

Practitioners should be aware that some individuals infected with the virus develop a mild or asymptomatic case of the disease. Approximately 30% of those infected have no signs or symptoms. Children with HBV are often asymptomatic. However, asymptomatic patients are just as infectious as those who are more symptomatic. Only a blood test will tell whether an individual is infected with HBV.

Fully 70% of the people who have recovered from the symptomatic stage of the disease are still infectious for three months or more after symptoms have subsided; 6% of individuals infected after age 5 are lifelong carriers.[13] One million people in the U.S. are chronic carriers of HBV.[14] These chronic carriers of the virus may develop cirrhosis of the liver and liver cancer; 15-25% of chronically infected people die from chronic liver disease.[15]

Obviously if a practitioner becomes infected with HBV, she/he may unknowingly transmit HBV to patients or office staff. Professionally and legally the ramifications of this form of transmission are enormous. High standards of office hygiene and clean needle technique will greatly reduce the risk of HBV infection for practitioners as well as patients. A practitioner with acute HBV should not practice during the infectious period.

13. http://www.cdc.gov/ncidod/diseases/hepatitis/b/fact.htm (April 14, 2002)

14. http://www.cdc.gov/ncidod/diseases/hepatitis/b/faqb.htm (April 14, 2002)

15. ibid footnote 7

## Treatment of HBV

Pharmaceuticals do exist to treat chronic hepatitis[16] but there is no biomedical treatment for persons infected with HBV other than treatment of the symptoms such as bed rest and reduced activity. In some cases, an injection with hepatitis B immune globulin (HBIG) immediately after exposure may provide protection to an unvaccinated person. The HBV vaccine series may also provide protection.

# Non-A, Non-B Hepatitis

## Hepatitis C (HCV)

Hepatitis C is the etiology of 40-60% of chronic liver disease in the U.S. HCV is known to be transmitted by exposure to contaminated blood and is principally found in adults. HCV is the most common form of transfusion-associated hepatitis. A large number of HCV infections appear among intravenous drug abusers. About one quarter of HIV-infected individuals in the U.S. are also infected with HCV. While there is no clear cut indication that HCV is transmitted via sexual contact independently of other risk factors, there is some evidence that sexual contact may be a mode of transmission of HCV with a low rate of transmission. Thus, while the transmission rate of HCV via sexual contact independent or other means of transmission is low, if it is in fact present, the serious health consequences of such transmission would make it important to view sexual transmission of HCV as a serious risk.[17, 18] There is no vaccine for HCV.

The incubation period of HCV is 20 to 90 days with most cases occurring 5 to 10 weeks after exposure. The period of communicability extends from one week after exposure through the chronic stage. The onset is insidious and accompanied by anorexia, nausea, vomiting, and jaundice. The course is similar to HBV but more prolonged. About half of HCV patients develop chronic hepatitis and many of these patients progress to develop cirrhosis and liver cancer. Therapy for hepatitis C is a rapidly changing area of clinical practice.

> The Surgeon General of the United States has urged people who may have had blood transfusions before July 1992 to be tested for hepatitis C.

## Hepatitis D (HDV)

HDV, sometimes known as Delta Hepatitis, is a defective virus that requires concurrent HBV infection for development of disease. In the U.S. most cases of hepatitis D occur in IV drug users and

---

16. A Consensus Development Conference Panel convened by the National Institutes of Health in 1997 recommended antiviral therapy for patients with chronic hepatitis C who are at greatest risk for progression to cirrhosis. Alpha interferon and lamivudine are two drugs licensed for the treatment of persons with chronic hepatitis B. These drugs are effective in up to 40% of patients.

17. 18 Yee LJ, Weiss HL, Langer RG, Hererra J, Kaslow RA, Leeuwen DJ, Risk factors for acquisition of hepatitis C virus infection: a case series and potential implications for disease surveillance, *BMC Infect Dis* 2001; 1:8

18. Stroffolini T, Lorenzoni U, Menniti-Ippolito F, Infantolino D, Chiaramonte M, Hepatitis C virus infection in spouses: sexual transmission or common exposure to the same risk factors? *Am J Gastroenterol.* 2001 Nov; 96(96):3051-3

hemophiliacs. There is no vaccine for HDV. However, since the HDV virus requires the presence of HBV, the vaccine against HBV is effective against HDV related disease.

The outcome of simultaneous HBV and HDV is no different from the outcome of HBV alone. However, when chronic HBV infection is accompanied by HDV, it may lead to severe, fulminating hepatitis or transform a mild or asymptomatic chronic HBV into a more severe disease process or accelerate its course.

### Hepatitis E

Hepatitis E is also known as epidemic non-A, non-B hepatitis and has occurred in large outbreaks in developing countries. HEV is rarely seen in the U.S. Most outbreaks have been linked to fecal contamination of the water supply. The incubation period is 15 to 60 days, with an average of 40 days. The time period of communicability is unknown. The disease is characterized by sudden onset of fever, malaise, nausea, and anorexia. The disease varies in severity from a mild illness lasting 7 to 14 days to a severely disabling disease lasting several months. Jaundice may be present. Pregnant women have a high (20%) mortality rate. There is no evidence of a chronic infection in long-term follow-up with patients with HEV. There is no vaccine for HEV.

## Chronic Carriers of Hepatitis

Chronic carriers are people who continue to shed hepatitis virus via bodily fluids and excretions long after infection. They are classified into two categories: Chronic Persistent and Chronic Active. A "Chronic Persistent" carrier is asymptomatic or has very minimal symptoms but can continue to infect others. A "Chronic Active" carrier has a progressive symptomatic disease that continues to damage the liver. Symptoms include malaise, weight loss, loss of appetite, and often jaundice.

Hepatitis A never becomes chronic. Hepatitis B becomes chronic in 5 to 10% of infections, HCV about 50% of the time. To get a good hepatitis history as part of the patient intake, ask about contact with blood products such as transfusions, dialysis, and injection drug use. Patients who have received transfusions or dialysis, or who have a history of injection drug use present a greater risk. Also, many patients in a public health care setting, such as chemical dependency, HIV, and TB clinics, have or have a history of some form of hepatitis, but may not know what type and may not know whether they are chronic carriers. This emphasizes the importance of obtaining a complete medical history and using universal precautions on every patient.

## Prevention of Hepatitis

One of the strongest reasons for the development of the clean needle technique protocol in 1984 was to provide guidelines to prevent the transmission of hepatitis within acupuncture clinic settings. This reason still exists today. Strict adherence to clean needle technique is essential in order to prevent transmission of HBV or a related virus to patients, practitioners, and staff.

## Summary of Hepatitis Characteristics

| Hepatitis | Incubation | Transmission | Onset | Vaccine | Chronic |
|-----------|-----------|--------------|-------|---------|---------|
| A | 15-50 days | Fecal-oral | Abrupt | Yes | No |
| B | 50-180 days | Bloodborne | Insidious | Yes | 5-10% |
| C | 20-90 days | Bloodborne | Insidious | No | 50% |
| D | Unknown | Unknown | Unknown | No | Unknown |
| E | 15-60 days | Fecal-oral | Abrupt | No | No |

# Human Immunodeficiency Disease (HIV)

## What Is HIV?

Two types of HIV have been identified: HIV-1 and HIV-2. Although they have similar epidemiological and pathological characteristics, they are different serologically and geographically. Generally, HIV targets the CD4(T4) lymphocyte as its host, which interrupts the cell-mediated response to antigens. HIV turns the CD4 (T4) lymphocyte into a reproduction factory that eventually destroys the cell once its replication duties have been performed. The CD4 (T4) cell count is finally reduced, producing an immune deficit from which the body cannot recover. Since the CD4 (T4) lymphocyte plays a crucial role in regulation of the immune system, its depletion due to HIV infection impacts the immune response.

HIV causes progressive damage to the human immune system over a variable period of time, making the individual vulnerable to a host of infections and malignancies. The condition known as Acquired Immune Deficiency Syndrome (AIDS) represents the late stage of HIV infection.

## HIV Transmission

Unlike HBV, there is no evidence to prove HIV is spread by any form of casual contact. Casual contact consists of any activity that does not involve the exchange of body fluids such as blood, semen, or vaginal secretions. Non-risk casual contact can include shaking hands, touching, hugging, holding hands, or casual kissing. Use of objects handled or touched by an HIV-infected person (for example, a telephone or toilet seat) has also not been shown to spread the virus.

### The Risk of HIV Transmission Through Invasive Procedures

In general, the risk for HIV transmission between patients and health care workers is very low.[19] Adherence to CDCP-recommended procedures for universal precautions reduces the risk to a negligible level. Practitioners should prevent direct blood contact and carry out proper cleaning and sterilization of instruments and other patient-care equipment.

---

19. As of June 30, 1999, a total of 191 U.S. workers had been reported to the CDCP's national surveillance system for occupationally acquired HIV infection. Beltrani et.al. *op.cite* p. 390

### Individuals at Risk of Infection With HIV

The first case of AIDS in the United States was reported in 1981. By the end of 1981, a total of 316 cases of this newly discovered disease were reported to the CDCP. Within five years (1986) the number had risen to 23,000, and by the spring of 1990, the number of reported cases of AIDS in the U.S. had reached 132,000. As of April 2002 the cumulative number of AIDS cases reported to CDC was over 793,000, of which almost 9,000 were reported in children under age 13. Total deaths of persons reported with AIDS were over 457,000, including over 5,000 children under age 15.[20] An estimated 15,000 people become infected worldwide every day.[21]

> Anyone in a profession with a high risk of blood exposure (such as health care workers) is in danger of contracting the virus which causes AIDS. Thus it is critical to use Universal Precautions with every patient.

It is important to note that the population distribution of HIV has changed. Initially HIV was found primarily among male homosexuals, IV drug users, sex workers, and transfusion recipients. Today HIV is no longer limited to these initial population groups. Recently, more cases have arisen due to unsafe sex between partners of different sexes and transplacental transmission. However, anyone who engages in 'at risk' behaviors (mainly unsafe sex with an infected partner and needle sharing) or is in a profession with a high risk of blood exposure (such as health care workers) is in danger of contracting the virus which causes AIDS. As of April 2002 CDC is aware of 57 health care workers in the United States who have been documented as having seroconverted to HIV following occupational exposures. Twenty-six have developed AIDS. These individuals who seroconverted include 19 laboratory workers (16 of whom were clinical laboratory workers), 24 nurses, 6 physicians, 2 surgical technicians, 1 dialysis technician, 1 respiratory therapist, 1 health aide, 1 embalmer/morgue technician, and 2 housekeeper/maintenance workers. The exposures were as follows: 48 had percutaneous (puncture/cut injury) exposure, 5 had mucocutaneous (mucous membrane and/or skin) exposure, 2 had both percutaneous and mucocutaneous exposure, and 2 had an unknown route of exposure. Forty-nine health care workers were exposed to HIV-infected blood, 3 to concentrated virus in a laboratory, 1 to visibly bloody fluid, and 4 to an unspecified fluid. CDC is also aware of 137 other cases of HIV infection or AIDS among health care workers who have not reported other risk factors for HIV infection and who report a history of occupational exposure to blood, body fluids, or HIV-infected laboratory material, but for whom seroconversion after exposure was not documented. The number of these workers who acquired their infection through occupational exposures is unknown.[22] It is critical to use universal precautions with every patient.

Because of the long incubation period of HIV (anywhere from 2 to 15 years from initial infection to onset of AIDS), the vast majority of HIV-infected individuals have no symptoms and may not know they are infected. However, anyone infected with HIV may be able to transmit the virus to others via

20.  www.cdc.gov/hiv (April 14, 2002)

21.  Gayle, HD and Hill, GL, "Global Impact of Human Immunodeficiency Virus and AIDS," *Clinical Microbiology Reviews* 14, No. 2 (April 2001) p. 327

22.  www.cdc.gov/hiv (April 14, 2002)

bodily fluids, including blood, semen, or vaginal secretions, regardless of whether or not they have developed symptoms of AIDS. It is critical that every practitioner bears this in mind during treatment. It is beneficial to routinely incorporate into the patient evaluation's risk assessment strategies to determine the likelihood of exposure to, or the presence of, HBV or HIV infection such as:

❖ Client's history regarding exposure to blood and blood products. ("Have you had a blood transfusion?")
❖ Client's history of drug use. ("What drugs have you used in the past ten years?")
❖ Client's sexual history/history of sexually transmitted diseases. ("How many sex partners have you had in the last two years?)"

### Testing for HIV/AIDS

Voluntary, anonymous testing is encouraged, especially for those who fall into the following categories:

❖ Persons in professions with a high-risk exposure.
❖ Persons who have had a sexually transmitted disease.
❖ Those who have used IV drugs and shared needles.
❖ Men who have had sex with other men since 1978.
❖ Men and women who have traded sex for money, food, drugs, or other items.
❖ People who have had multiple sex partners and used intravenous injected drugs.
❖ Sexual or needle-sharing partners of the above.
❖ Any woman thinking of becoming pregnant.

For specific information on locations and requirements on testing for HIV, check with the local health department.

### Reporting of HIV/AIDS

A uniform case definition and case report form is now used in all fifty states for the reporting of diagnosed cases of AIDS. Revisions in the definition of clinical AIDS have broadened the range of AIDS-indicator diseases and conditions. Using HIV diagnostic tests has improved the sensitivity and specificity of the definition.

## The HIV Infection Process

Infection with HIV can present a continuum ranging from asymptomatic to symptomatic (exhibiting one or more of the symptoms associated with impaired immune function) to AIDS (having the set of symptoms associated with the specifically defined syndrome).

Initial HIV infection is usually followed within 2 to 4 weeks by a febrile illness resembling mononucleosis or influenza which resolves spontaneously and which many people do not note as significant at the time. Some people infected with HIV remain relatively healthy for many years before the symptoms of HIV infection appear. Scientists have estimated that about half of the people with HIV develop AIDS within 10 years after becoming infected.

As the immune damage progresses, the most common symptoms are fever, malaise, body aches, maculopapular rash, lymphadenopathy, and headache. Other symptoms include persistent fever and night sweats; rapid, unexplained loss of weight; chronic diarrhea not explained by other causes; persistent cough that is not from smoking or the flu, and flat or raised, pigmented lesions on the skin ranging in color from faint pink to red, brown, or blue. Many of these symptoms are non-specific and are seen in many other conditions.

Data indicates that most people infected with HIV eventually develop AIDS. These individuals develop opportunistic infections and neoplastic disorders rarely seen in individuals with a healthy immune system. These infections include candidiasis, cytomegalovirus, Kaposi's sarcoma, and Pneumocystis carinii pneumonia, which is the most common opportunistic infection and cause of death in AIDS patients.

The clinical presentations of AIDS patients vary extensively. Individuals may present with HIV "wasting disease," which is characterized by severe, involuntary weight loss, chronic diarrhea, constant or intermittent weakness, and fever for 30 days or longer. If HIV infects cells in the cerebrospinal fluid, individuals may develop HIV encephalopathy, myelopathy, peripheral neuropathy, or dementia with symptoms ranging from apathy and depression to memory loss and motor dysfunction and death.[23]

Presently it is not known why some people infected with the virus develop symptoms more quickly than others do. Researchers have proposed that certain co-factors such as stress, poor nutrition, alcohol or drug abuse, and certain sexually transmitted diseases (STDs), such as syphilis, may trigger the virus to begin replicating.

## Treatment of HIV

AIDS represents the critical stage of the clinical spectrum of HIV infection. At the present time there is no cure or vaccine for AIDS, although a variety of drugs are being used to slow the progression of the disease and treat some of the opportunistic infections.

An additional risk to practitioners working with persons with HIV is that some of the common secondary infections in this population are themselves contagious. These include tuberculosis, staphylococcus, herpes, and hepatitis. Appropriate precautions should be taken in such cases: use of masks in case of respiratory infection and gloves in case of skin infection.

# PROTECTION OF PATIENTS, PRACTITIONERS, AND STAFF

Blood-to-blood contact is the most direct method of transmitting HBV and HIV. When infected blood enters the bloodstream of another person, the chances of acquiring these viruses are

---

23. CDCP HIV/AIDS Update, www.cdc.gov (November 2001)

extremely high. In the health care workplace, the risk of infection from exposure to contaminated blood is much greater for HBV than HIV. The most typical mode of transmission is percutaneous exposure that occurs from contaminated instruments (mostly from needlesticks), or contact of contaminated blood with non-intact skin. The risk, however, is extremely low if universal precautions are followed. Universal precautions, as defined by the CDCP, include the use of gloves, masks, gowns, goggles, and prevention techniques appropriate to the particular health care setting.

CHAPTER 2

# CNT Protocols

IT HAS BEEN DETERMINED THAT occupational exposure to bloodborne pathogens poses a significant risk to health care workers. This exposure can be eliminated or greatly reduced through work practice habits, personal protection, training, vaccination, labeling, and medical surveillance.[24] Therefore, two federal agencies have established standards that apply to all medical practitioners, including licensed acupuncturists. The CDCP set procedures that are to be followed with regard to occupational exposure to bloodborne pathogens in health care settings in the United States. These procedures are known as "Universal Precautions." OSHA has codified the CDCP standards into recommendations that apply to all health care providers. The NAF has utilized these guidelines and recommendations, in addition to the medical community's standard procedures for giving injections and feedback from the acupuncture community, in developing the CNT protocols. It is important to remember that the application of CNT in a clinical setting is a thoughtful process based on an understanding of principles rather than a rote application of memorized guidelines.

## BASIC PRINCIPLES OF CNT

Clean needle technique includes the following basic elements:

➡ Always wash hands between patients.
➡ Always use sterile needles.
➡ Always establish a clean field.
➡ Always wash hands just prior to inserting needles if hands have been contaminated.
➡ Always immediately isolate used needles.

---

24. For copies of the OSHA standards contact: OSHA Publications, U.S. Department of Labor/OSHA, PO Box 37535, Washington, D.C. 20013, 202/693-1888.

Besides the obvious necessity for sterile needles, public health agencies identify handwashing as the single most important action in preventing cross-infection. Hands should be washed with soap under running water immediately after leaving each patient and just prior to the insertion of a needle if one's hands have been contaminated by actions such as adjusting patient's clothing, answering the telephone and touching hair.

> The main goal of universal precautions is the prevention of exposure and prevention of disease if exposure occurs.

Contaminated needles are the greatest source of risk to the practitioner and patient. It is essential to minimize handling used needles during disposal or until after they have been sterilized. These basic principles will be discussed in the sections that follow.

It is essential to be meticulous in following all aspects of clean needle technique protocol and universal precautions. This includes the use of sterile needles, handwashing between treatments, and isolation of used needles. Skin and mucus membrane contacts frequently can be prevented with the use of barrier precautions such as gloves, masks, gowns and goggles. However, the greatest risk of blood-borne pathogen transmission comes from needlestick injuries. These are not prevented by barriers but instead require strict adherence to CNT protocols by practitioners, the continuing recognition of the need to handle all patients as if they were potentially infectious and the need to train all staff in clean needle protocols and universal precautions.

Precautions are the same for hepatitis and AIDS as well as for other diseases that might be transmitted by violation of clean procedure and needlestick accidents. Health care workers are advised to develop standard, habitual procedures for all patients that provide the necessary protection against cross-infection.

# CATEGORIES FOR CLEAN AND SAFE PRACTICE

The standard in the United States is that any instrument that penetrates the skin or is brought into contact with mucous membranes or a sterile field must be sterile. This manual presents step-by-step protocols to help develop practical office procedures that ensure clean and safe practice.

Throughout this manual, the NAF recommendations for clean and safe practice are noted in italics and given in three categories as follows:

*Critical:* This addresses the area of highest clinical risk. The protocol is considered essential for the safety of the patient and practitioner, and omission could constitute a serious public health risk.

*Strongly Recommended:* These measures are strongly supported by clinical studies that show their effectiveness in reducing risk or are viewed as important by the majority of epidemiologists. They are considered essential measures and frequently address areas of high clinical risk.

*Recommended:* These measures include two types of recommendations: those that are supported by highly suggestive, but perhaps less generalizable, clinical studies in a related field, and those that have not been adequately researched, but have a strong theoretical rationale indicating that they might be very effective for clean and safe practice. Both types are judged to be practical to implement but are not considered essential practice for every practitioner in every situation. They should, however, be considered by practitioners for implementation into their practices.

# DEFINITIONS

The following is a list of definitions of terms that are frequently used in this section of the *CNT Manual.*

*Sterilization:* The use of procedures that destroy all microbial life, including viruses. This is a rigid, uncompromising term. There is no such thing as partial sterility. In acupuncture, sterilization is required for all instruments that pierce the skin (needles, plum-blossom needles, etc.) or those items that may come into contact with instruments that pierce the skin (storage trays, forceps, guide tubes for needles, etc.)

*Contamination:* The introduction of disease-causing agents into or onto previously clean or sterile objects, making them impure or unclean.

*Aseptic techniques:* Techniques for preventing infection during invasive procedures such as surgical operations, dressing wounds, or procedures involving a puncture of the skin (e.g., injections, acupuncture). Aseptic techniques vary for different types of invasive procedures. The level of aseptic technique necessary for surgery is not necessary for acupuncture.

*Antiseptic:* Products designed to reduce the density of microbial life on living tissue, particularly on the skin of the patient or practitioner.

*Disinfection:* The use of chemicals and procedures designed to destroy or reduce the number of pathogens on inanimate objects such as equipment and clinic surfaces. It must be recognized that some bacteria, spores, and viruses may resist the often lethal effects of many chemicals.

*Disinfectants:* The chemicals employed in disinfection. They should only be used on inanimate objects, and are not to be confused with antiseptics that are applied to the body.

*Clean technique:* The use of techniques (antisepsis, disinfection, sterilization, washing, etc.) designed to reduce the risk of infection of patients, practitioners, and office personnel by killing or reducing the strength of pathogens, thereby reducing the chances for contact between the pathogens and the patients and personnel.

*Clean field:* The area that has been prepared to contain the equipment necessary for acupuncture, in such a way as to protect the sterility of the needles. By extension, this includes not only the clean surface on which equipment will be placed, but also the patient's skin around the selected acupuncture points, and anything that touches the skin.

# RECOMMENDATIONS FOR PRACTITIONERS

## Yearly Physical

*It is recommended that health care professionals have a yearly physical that includes testing for tuberculosis (PPD type).*

## Clothing

*It is recommended that acupuncturists wear clean, washable or disposable protective clothing while performing treatments. The fabric should be chosen to avoid trapping and shedding contaminating particles or infectious agents in the clean field. Loose or large jewelry, clothing, and hairstyles that touch the client or break the clean field should be avoided.*

## Hand Care

Acupuncturists must take great care to maintain the cleanliness of their hands, keeping the nails short. Hand cleanliness is a part of clean needle technique. *It is strongly recommended that all cuts and wounds on the practitioner's hands be washed and dressed immediately for the protection of both patient and practitioner.* All cuts, wounds, abrasions, chapped hands, hang nails, torn cuticles, etc. must be covered with rubber gloves or finger cots. Rubber gloves and finger cots need not be sterile.

## Personal Health

An acupuncturist who is suffering from an infectious disease can transmit the disease to his or her client in various ways. Appropriate medical attention should be sought for infectious diseases.

In its guidelines, the American Hospital Association recommends: "Patient care personnel having overt clinical infection, such as streptococcal pharyngitis (strep throat), active influenza, or a staphylococcal furuncle (boil), should restrict themselves from patient contact. Personnel with minor infections of the skin and minor viral infections of the upper respiratory tract may work so long as they are scrupulous in their practice of personal hygiene."[25]

## Testing for TB, HBV, HCV and HIV

*TB Testing:* In addition to a yearly physical, the CDCP suggests that practitioners who work in an inner city clinic, with AIDS patients or drug addicts, have a PPD test every six months. The CDCP does not recommend that health care workers who work in a low risk setting receive a TB vaccination. "The transmission of TB is a recognized risk in health care settings and is of particular concern in settings where HIV-infected persons work, volunteer, visit, or receive care.

---

25.  Iippolito, et. al., "The Risk of Occupational Human Immunodeficiency Virus Infection in Health Care Workers," Arch *Intern Med* 153 (1993), 1456.

Effective TB infection-control programs should be implemented in health-care facilities and other institutional settings (e.g. shelters for homeless persons and correctional facilities)."[26] HCWs who perform exposure-prone procedures should know their HBV or HIV antibody status.

*HBV Testing:* Various tests for HBV can detect either the presence of the virus itself or antibodies to the virus. Testing for evidence of hepatitis B infection should be routine for medical practitioners, especially those with occupational exposure potential. Hospitals and blood banks are required to test for HBV with a very sensitive test that identifies HBV antigen markers.

*HCV Testing:* Generally, the initial laboratory test for HCV is to determine if the person has antibodies to the virus. If the test is positive, it means that the person has been exposed to the virus and may or may not have active hepatitis C. Additional testing will need to be done to determine if the person is a carrier, has chronic hepatitis or is immune.

*HIV Testing:* Generally the initial laboratory test that is done for HIV is a test for HIV antibodies. This test can help determine if the person has been infected with the virus but can not determine the stage of disease. There are rapid HIV tests that can provide results within 1 hour of testing. A positive test should be confirmed with a western blot or IFA (immunoflourescent assay) test.

Health care workers (HCWs) who are infected with HIV or HBV should not perform exposure-prone procedures unless they have received counseling from an expert review panel regarding the circumstances under which they may continue to perform these procedures. The review panel should include experts who represent a balanced perspective and might include all of the following: (a) the HCW's personal physician, (b) an infectious disease specialist with expertise in the epidemiology of HIV and HBV transmission, (c) a health professional with expertise in the procedures performed by the HCW, and (d) state or local public health officials. If the HCW is institution-based, the panel could include the hospital epidemiologist or other infection-control staff. HCWs based outside the hospital/ institutional setting should seek advice from appropriate state and local public health officials regarding the review process. It goes without saying that such panels would be required to observe the confidentiality and privacy rights of infected HCWs.

❖ Infected HCWs should notify prospective patients of their seropositive status before undertaking exposure-prone invasive procedures.

❖ Mandatory testing of HCWs for HIV antibodies, HBsAg, or HBeAg is not recommended. The risk is not sufficient to justify the costs such mandatory testing programs would incur.

Education, training, and appropriate confidentiality safeguards are the best means to insure HCW compliance with recommended prevention procedures

---

26.  Centers for Disease Control and Prevention, Immunization of Health-Care workers: Recommendations of the Advisory Committee on Immunization Practices (ACIP) and the Hospital Infection Control Practices Advisory Committee (HICPAC), MMR 1997; 46 (No. RR18).

# RECOMMENDATIONS FOR EQUIPMENT

## Acupuncture Needles

*It is critical that all acupuncture needles and instruments that penetrate the skin be sterile for each insertion.*[27] This includes acupuncture needles, plum-blossom or seven-star needles, and any other equipment that might break the skin.

*It is critical that acupuncture be performed with filiform (solid) acupuncture needles.* The round polished points of acupuncture needles are easy to clean and do minimal damage to the skin and flesh when they penetrate. Hollow medical injection needles are not recommended because they have a cutting edge and cause more tissue damage. In addition, they may catch blood or tissue in the hollow shaft. Stainless steel is the material of choice for acupuncture needles since softer metals are more likely to pit, corrode, tarnish, or break.

*It is recommended to use disposable needles in an acupuncture practice.* The use of disposable needles is a good precaution because it decreases risk from equipment failure or human error. The use of disposable needles, however, does not solve all problems relating to safety and clean needle practices. The following still require careful attention:

1. *Packaging must be appropriate.* Some bubble-type packages loosen around the edges so that contamination becomes possible. Packaging that binds the needles too tightly increases risk of contamination in the struggle to free the needles. Avoid these types of packaging. Packages that have been bent, have a broken seal or show evidence of moisture damage should be discarded.

   Needles in soft plastic bags must be carried in a hard-sided container, and the individual packets must be handled carefully to avoid the needles puncturing the plastic from the inside and becoming contaminated by external contact.

2. *Needles must be removed from the sterile packaging in such a way as to avoid contamination.* For example, when opening the packet, that part that has been touched by the fingers must be folded back to avoid contact with the needle. Special care is needed with multiple-needle packages if one needle is removed at a time.

*It is strongly recommended that practitioners who use reusable needles use the double sterilization procedures outlined in this manual.*

*It is also recommended that when using reusable needles, new needles be used for each new patient and then used only for that patient, sterilizing after each use.* This system may alleviate any concerns regarding cross-infection. Several systems available from medical supply houses allow practitioners to isolate patients' needles in individual packets for autoclaving and to label and store them properly.

---

27. Issues in Healthcare Settings "Sterilization or Disinfection of Medical Devices: General Principles", *Division of Healthcare Quality Promotion*, CDC 6/6/00.

## Needle Guide Tubes

*It is strongly recommended that needle guide tubes be sterile for each patient.* If sterilizable, guide tubes must be sterilized after each patient. If not sterilizable they should be disposed of after each patient.

## Needle Trays

*It is strongly recommended that all needle trays and gauze that contain sterile needles themselves be sterile.* Reusable needle trays should be sterilized between uses; disposable needle trays and gauze should be discarded after one use.

## Seven-Star or Plum-blossom Needles

*It is critical that reusable seven-star or plum-blossom needles be sterilized after each patient following the standard procedure. Disposable and plastic equipment that can not be sterilized must be used on only one patient.*

## Cupping Devices

It is strongly recommended that cupping devices be able to be autoclaved or sterilized in a chemical disinfectant bath. Since cupping should not be done over areas in which there are sores or lesions, as a general rule there is little likelihood of exposure to blood. If no bleeding occurs, cupping devices should be washed with soap and water between patients. However, if bleeding occurs, cupping devices must be able to be sterilized.

When breaking the seal on a cup, use caution due to the potential formation of aerosols when the vacuum is broken. Where there is blood or other body fluids in the cupped area, breaking the vacuum seal may result in the aerosol containing infectious material.

CHAPTER **3**

# Applying CNT in an Acupuncture Treatment

## GENERAL GUIDELINES

### Establishing a Clean Work Area

An acupuncturist's office should be kept clean, tidy, and as free as possible from dirt and dust. OSHA requires that the workplace be maintained in a clean and sanitary condition and that there is an appropriate written schedule for cleaning and decontamination. The cleanliness of the general environment also has a direct impact on the practitioner's ability to create a clean field and maintain the sterility of the needles. If a contractor is responsible for clinic maintenance, the contractor must be instructed regarding maintenance and the presence of biohazardous materials.

A sink with hot and cold running water must be located in or near the treatment rooms.

Bar soap is not recommended because of the risk of bacterial growth and contamination of the sludge from melted soap. Reusable containers of liquid soap should be washed thoroughly and allowed to dry before refilling with fresh soap.

Single use, disposable towels should be used to dry the hands. Clean paper towels are appropriate. Cloth towels are not.

Any paper or other disposable material used as a covering on a chair, seat or couch, and any towel, cloth, sheet, gown, or other article that is applied to the patient's skin should be clean, and should not previously have been used in connection with any other patient unless laundered after use.

> Hepatitis B can survive on surfaces for at least one week at room temperature.

The treatment tabletops, shelves and other working surfaces should have a smooth, impervious surface, be in good repair, and be cleaned with a suitable disinfectant at least once a day and whenever visibly contaminated or whenever a patient may have contaminated the surface, for example, by profuse sweating.

*Disinfectants are recommended for office surfaces and equipment.* Disinfectants do not kill all germs or spores, but they will reduce the danger of infection. Clorox, Lysol and Microquat are common disinfectants that neutralize most viruses, including hepatitis B. (There are also many others.) These solutions lose strength over time and must be remade at specified intervals. They cannot be stored indefinitely. Check with the manufacturer for expiration times. Also, the solutions must be made according to manufacturer's instructions. The manufacturer's suggested concentrations must be strictly followed. Disinfectants must be labeled if not in the original bottle. The label should state what the solution is, when it was mixed and the concentration.

Used disinfectants must be carefully poured down the sink or toilet and flushed with running water since they become contaminated with use.

## Positioning the Patient

In order to make the patient comfortable and facilitate location of points, the patient should be placed in a posture suitable to the points selected. If the patient is kept in an awkward posture, undue fatigue or fainting may occur. There is also a possibility of accidents such as a needle bending or breaking if the patient changes position abruptly. Usually the supine position is desir-

> The best way to reduce occupational risk of infection is to follow universal precautions.

able when needling the points of the frontal and facial regions, chest and abdomen, and the anterior or lateral aspect of the lower extremities. A prone position is preferable for occipital, neck, lumbo-dorsal regions and the posterior aspect of the lower extremities, while lateral recumbent position facilitates needling of points on the lateral aspect of the body. For the points on the head, back and upper extremities, a comfortable sitting position is also suitable.

## Handwashing

According to the Centers for Disease Control in Atlanta, hand-washing is the most important single procedure for preventing infection in a health care setting. Handwashing has been shown to eliminate or markedly reduce pathogenic organisms on the hand.

> Health care workers must assume all patients are infected with HBV or HIV, thus taking adequate non-discriminatory precautions to protect themselves.

Most routine activities involving direct patient contact, e.g., taking pulses or blood pressure or shaking hands do not in themselves require handwashing. But the hands should always be washed just before the actual acupuncture procedure.

Washing hands in preparation for a medical procedure is a very different process than washing hands before a meal. Here is a breakdown of the steps for handwashing:

1.  Gather the equipment needed to wash hands: paper towels, soap, and running water. Liquid soap is recommended due to the risk of contamination when using bar soap.

2.  Roll up long sleeves, remove watch and jewelry, if applicable. A plain ring like a wedding band is acceptable, but bulky jewelry or rings with stones or intricate work should be removed. (Jewelry can harbor infectious agents in crevices that are not easily accessible.)

3.  Wet the soap and hands thoroughly.

4.  Rub the soap to make lather.

5.  Wash the entire surface of the hands between the fingers, around and under the fingernails and up to above the wrist.

6.  Run water over the hands again to clean them.

7.  Lower the hands so that water and soap drain off the fingertips as they are rinsed.

8.  Soap and repeat the washing process.

9.  Give the hands a final rinse.

10. Turn off the tap with a towel or use an elbow so that hands do not become soiled. Do not dry hands with the towel used to turn off the tap.

11. Dry the hands carefully using a clean paper towel or shake the hands dry in the air.

Particular attention should be paid to fingernails, which should be kept short and clean.

There are two types of infectious agents on the skin: resident and transient. Transient agents include those that are picked up from one patient and possibly carried to another. Soap is adequate for cleansing the surface of the skin of this type of infectious agent. Resident agents, which lodge deeper in the skin, present additional risk for an immuno-compromised patient and germicidal soap or an alcohol-based hand disinfectant should be used. *Therefore it is strongly recommended that antimicrobial products be used for washing before and after treating patients who are severely immunocompromised* (e.g., those with HIV or who are undergoing chemotherapy or dialysis.)

Standard medical protocols for giving injections call for washing the hands before the procedure, palpating the area before swabbing it, and then inserting the needle.[28]

*It is strongly recommended that acupuncturists always wash their hands:*

1.  *Immediately before the acupuncture procedure*

2.  *After contact with blood or body fluids or obvious environmental contaminants*

3.  *At the end of a treatment.* [29,30]

4.  *Whenever their hands become contaminated during a treatment.*

Handwashing with disinfecting soap and running water is the most effective form of handwashing. However, when there is no sink available, practitioners may use an alcohol-based hand disinfectant.

---

28. Standard nursing procedure also recommends using gloves for any injection, whether it is intra-muscular or intra-venous. Potter, *Fundamentals of Nursing* (5th edition, 2001).

29. "APIC Guidelines for Handwashing and Hand Antisepsis in Health-Care Settings", *American Journal of Infection Control* 23:251-269 (1995).

30. Weinstein, Robert A., *Controlling Antimicrobial Resistance in Hospitals: Infection Control and Use of Antibiotics*, Emerging Infectious Diseases, Vol. 7, No.2, Mar-Apr 2001.

An alcohol-based hand disinfectant can degerm hands in less than 30 seconds and enhance killing of transient hand flora without the use of running water, soap and hand-drying facilities.[31] Alcohol-based hand disinfectants actually improve skin condition, presumably because they contain emollients. Studies have shown that clinicians find them convenient, accessible and less irritating to the skin.[32] CDCP has also accepted the use of antiseptic hand cleansers or towelettes. [33]

The necessity of handwashing between patients and the use of universal precautions reflects the importance of treating all patients as if they were carriers of hepatitis or HIV. Beyond this, the need to wash the hands is based on whether the hands become contaminated during the course of treatment.

Practitioners who treat one patient and then return to remove the needles after inserting needles in another patient should wash their hands between each such contact with each patient.

*If the hands are contaminated after washing, it is strongly recommended that the fingertips be cleansed before the next step, whether it be palpating the acupuncture point or inserting the needle.* Infectious agents are on every non-sterile surface. Of these, staphylococcus is perhaps the most serious contaminant found on the skin and on other surfaces.

Assuming that the practitioner's hands were washed after the last treatment, examples of potential contamination before the next treatment include the practitioner touching his/her face, hair, or eyes or using a pen (which has been handled before, during and after treatments for weeks at a time), helping the patient adjust clothing or remove shoes, picking up dropped items from the floor and answering the telephone.

> Universal precautions should apply to blood, body fluids containing visible blood, semen, vaginal secretions, tissues, cerebrospinal fluid, synovial fluid, pleural fluid, peritoneal fluid, pericardial fluid, and amniotic fluid.

Cleansing the fingertips of the wide variety of potential contaminants is a significant measure for reducing the risk of infection. Swabbing with alcohol or using an alcohol-based hand rub, germicidal scrub or antiseptic towelette is an acceptable substitute for a full handwashing at this stage.

---

31.  http://www.cdc.gov/ncidod/eid/vol7no2/weinstein.htm.

32.  Boyce, JM, et al., Proceedings of the 9th Annual Society for Healthcare Epidemiology of America Meeting, April 18-20, 1999, San Francisco, CA.

33.  See *CFR* 56, No. 235 (December 1991) 64116 -17 which discusses OSHA's decision "to accept the use of alternative handwashing methods as an interim measure when soap and water are not a feasible means of handwashing." This includes the use of antiseptic hand cleansers or towelettes. However, "hands shall be washed with soap and running water as soon as feasible." OSHA also goes on to clarify that hands "are not the only body area that needs to be washed upon contamination but also any other skin or mucous membrane which has had contact with blood or other potentially infectious materials." See also APIC Guidelines *op. cite.*

## Preparing the Site for Insertion of a Needle

*It is strongly recommended that practitioners check that the skin areas to be treated are free of any cuts, wounds, or diseases.* Acupuncture needles should never be inserted through inflamed, irritated, diseased, or broken skin. Otherwise, infections can be carried directly into the body past the broken skin barrier.

*It is strongly recommended that practitioners ensure that the part of the body to be treated is clean.*[34] The areas to be needled should be cleaned with an alcohol-impregnated swab.[35] If body parts (e.g., the feet) are grossly dirty, they should be washed first with soap and water, then swabbed as needed with an alcohol swab.

According to CDCP, 70% isopropyl alcohol is adequate for preparing a patient's skin for procedures such as inserting needles. Ninety-percent isopropyl alcohol is unacceptable because it evaporates too quickly to have an antiseptic effect. Other cleaning agents, if used, should also have adequate antiseptic properties. Iodophor such as Betadyne followed by alcohol swab or benzylconium chloride is recommended for immunocompromised patients.

Swab the points and allow the alcohol to dry. *It is recommended that points be swabbed in a way that touches the area only once so as not to recontaminate the area.* One medical practice is to swab points using a rotary scrubbing motion, spiraling out from the center. Others are to swab from one end of the area to another or in a wide "C" motion. The same swab may be used for points in the same general area, for example, for several points on the back or on a single extremity such as the left forearm. A new swab should be used when changing areas of the body, for example from points on the torso to points on the extremities, or if the swab begins to change color.

The alcohol should be allowed to dry to reduce discomfort on needling and to reduce the possibility of injecting minute amounts of contaminants suspended in the alcohol.

## Palpating the Point

It is acceptable clean technique to touch the acupuncture point after cleaning the skin, as long as the hands have not been contaminated. *However, it is strongly recommended that before picking up the needle or palpating the point, the hands should be washed again or the fingers should be swabbed with alcohol or an antimicrobial scrub if they have been contaminated since the last handwashing by arranging clothing, taking notes, etc.* (Swabbing is acceptable for the second handwashing if there is not a sink in the treatment room.) After this second cleaning of the fingers, nothing should be touched but the needle handle, guide tube and the skin over the point. If anything else is touched, the fingers should be cleaned again before proceeding.

---

34.  It should be noted that although it is standard medical protocol to swab an area with alcohol prior to injecting a needle, there is some disagreement with this recommendation.

35.  The use of alcohol swabs is recommended rather than cotton balls and a pump-action alcohol dispenser.

## Using Sterile Needles

*It is critical that the needle shaft be maintained in a sterile state prior to insertion.* After removal from the packaging, nothing nonsterile must touch the shaft of the needle prior to insertion: neither the practitioner's hands nor other unsterile inanimate objects or surfaces. If the needle shaft is contaminated before insertion, it must be resterilized before use or discarded appropriately.

When opening a needle packet, the needles may be handled in any way that protects them from contact with anything that is not sterile. The packet should be opened and folded back in such a way that when the needles are removed, their shafts do not touch the part of the packet that was touched by the fingers while opening the packet.

*Needle insertion and manipulation must be performed without the practitioner's bare hands coming into contact with the shaft of the needle.* If the needle shaft must be supported, a *sterile* gauze pad or cotton ball is used. Support with *clean* gauze or cotton ball increases the risk of contamination and is not acceptable. The level of contamination introduced by the bare fingers on the needle shaft is also unacceptable since the skin, even immediately after washing or swabbing, may continue to shed viruses or other resident or transient infectious agents that could be pathogenic.

If the needle needs to be laid down after removal from the tray and prior to use, this can only be done on a surface that is known to be sterile, e.g., a sterile gauze pad.

When placing sterile objects on the sterile gauze pad, it is important to position them in such a way that the handle, which the practitioner touched, is set on the *clean* field, while the sterile portion (e.g. needle shafts or tips of tweezers) is on the *sterile* gauze.

## Using Guide Tubes

*It is strongly recommended that guide tubes be sterile at the beginning of each treatment on each patient.* Guide tubes may be used repeatedly on the same patient during the treatment, but must be resterilized before use on another patient.

According to the CDCP, it is critical that all objects that normally touch sterile tissue be sterile. While insertion tubes do not themselves break the skin, they touch the needle shaft, which does break the skin. Technically, the guide tube loses its sterility after it has touched the patient's skin and the practitioner's finger. But since both these contact points have been wiped with alcohol immediately before the contact, and since so little of the needle shaft actually touches the tube, it is considered acceptable to use the tube repeatedly on the same patient.

If a guide tube is used, dropping the needle into the tube handle first will reduce the risk of contaminating the point of the needle.

If guide tubes are used, they should be placed on the clean field between uses, since they have been handled and are no longer sterile.

# Using Gloves

*It is recommended that a rubber glove be used when there is risk of contact with blood or other potentially infectious body fluids. The use of gloves is not necessary during routine acupuncture practice in the absence of significant bleeding.*

The decision by an acupuncturist regarding whether gloves should be used must be viewed within the context of current research regarding risk factors involved in transmission of HBV and HIV and how these risk factors relate to both patients and practitioners within an acupuncture practice.

When discussing the risk of transmission of HBV to health care workers, OSHA noted that transmission "was related to the degree of blood exposure or frequency of needle exposure, and not to patient contact per se."[36] In 1992 the Center for Disease Control stated that, "No case of [HIV] infection due to casual contact with these fluids [sweat, tears, saliva] has been documented. Rather infection can occur only if infectious fluids enter the body either through a percutaneous or mucosal route."[37]

> In deciding whether to use gloves, practitioners must assess whether it can *"reasonably be anticipated"* that there will be contact with blood.

One common percutaneous method of transmission in a health care setting is through a needlestick. Although there is only one reported case of health care workers or patient HIV seroconversion reported after contact with either an acupuncture needle or a suture needle (a solid, filiform needle similar to acupuncture needles),[38] there are several reports of transmission of HIV to health care workers through contaminated hypodermic needles.[39] There are also reported cases of HBV seroconversion after contact with a contaminated acupuncture needle.[40] However, as noted by OSHA, gloving will not stop direct puncture injuries.[41] Only proper handling of contaminated needles will do that.

It is important to emphasize that gloves present a barrier only to blood and other potentially infectious fluids. Gloves offer no protection from an accidental needle stick, and if improperly used may actually increase the risk of accidental needle stick during an acupuncture procedure.[42]

Transmission may also occur through mucous membranes or skin. OSHA notes that splashes of

---

36. *CFR* 56, No. 235 (December 6, 1991) 64011 - 12. OSHA also noted that the factors in transmission of HBV from HCWs to patients were routine occurrence of significant blood exposure, trauma, and use of sharp instruments

37. Ibid. 64032.

38. Lao, Li Xing, "Safety Issues in Acupuncture," *Journal of Alternative Medicine,* 2. No. 1 (Spring 1996).

39. Ibid.

40. Beltrami, E.M. et. al, *Clinical Microbiology Reviews,* July 2000, pp. 385-407..

41. *Ibid.*

42. It should be noted that some practitioners feel that use of gloves during insertion of needles increases the risk of a needlestick due to clumsiness caused by the gloves.

blood or serum into the eye or mouth in clinical settings or laboratory settings must be regarded as potentially serious exposures and that blood and other infectious fluids may enter the body through small cuts on the skin.[43] However, the research shows that the risk of blood contact increases with the amount of blood involved in the procedure[44] and that the risk of seroconversion varies with the amount of blood to which the HCW is exposed. The risk of seroconversion increases if the exposure involves a larger quantity of blood, the source patient had a terminal illness or use of appropriate post-exposure treatment.

Each practitioner must consider these factors when assessing whether or not to use gloves. As noted earlier, standard nursing procedure recommends using gloves for any injection, whether it is intramuscular or intravenous.[45, 46] According to the OSHA Bloodborne Pathogens Standard, gloving is recommended when there will be contact with "other potentially infectious materials (OPIM), mucous membranes, and non-intact skin; when performing vascular access procedures and when handling or touching contaminated items or surfaces."[46]

In response to a query regarding auricular acupuncture for chemical dependency, one OSHA office has stated, "Since there is no exposure to blood or OPIM at the point of placing five acupuncture needles just under the surface of the skin in each ear, it is not necessary to wear gloves for that procedure. If there is reasonable anticipation that the employee may have hand contact with blood when the needles are removed, it would be necessary to wear gloves. On the other hand, if no blood contact with the employee's hand is reasonably anticipated during a procedure, gloves need not be worn."[47]

Thus, each practitioner must assess for him and herself the possibility of blood contact during each acupuncture treatment and act accordingly. Use of gloves is consistent with universal precautions recommended by disease control experts and provides the best protection for both practitioner and patient when there is the presence of potentially infectious material.

*In order to protect the practitioner, the use of gloves is strongly recommended in the following instances:*

➡ *During procedures such as bleeding where there is a greater risk of contact with larger amounts of blood.*

➡ *When working with patients who have open lesions or weeping exudates from their skin.*

➡ *When the practitioner has cuts, abrasions, chapped skin, hang nails or broken cuticles on his or her hand and the lesions are located in a location where they pose a hazard.*

-------

43. *CFR*, 56, No. 235 (December 6, 1991), 64010.

44. One study noted that the risk of a surgeon contacting blood increased when the patients blood loss greater than 250 cc's. Mary Rodts and Daniel Benson, "HIV Precautions for Prevention in the Workplace," *Orthopaedic Nursing* 11 No. 5 (September/October, 1992), 52-3.

45. Potter, *op. cite.*

46. 29 *CFR* 1910.1030 (d)(3)(ix).

47. Letter from Gilbert J. Saulter, Regional Administrator, OSHA Administration, Dallas, Texas, November 25, 1994.

➡ *When palpating or needling in the mouth or genital area.*

*In accord with OSHA requirements, it is strongly recommended that "disposable (single use) gloves (such as surgical or examination gloves) shall be replaced as soon as practical when contaminated, or as soon as feasible if they are torn, punctured, or when their ability to function as a barrier is compromised."* [48]

## Inserting Needle to Correct Depth

There is no absolute standard for the depth of acupuncture needling. Following are some general guidelines and recommendations:

1. Follow the suggested needle depths and angles of insertion indicated in major texts, being sure to allow for variation in body size. For instance, in puncturing the point CV 12 (Zhongwan), a strong sensation may be obtained when a depth of 0.5 inch is reached in a thin patient. On the other hand, sensation may only be induced when the needle is inserted further for an obese patient. Clinical, careful analysis should be made of each patient. For children, needle depths should be less than for an adult. Slow penetration allows the practitioners to sense changes in resistance and "arrival of Qi," which helps serve as a guide in adjusting the depth of insertion to body size.

2. In the thoracic and back regions, muscles are sometimes thin and important viscera, such as the heart, lungs, liver and spleen, are in close proximity. It is advisable to puncture cautiously, preferably at an appropriate angle as indicated in standard texts.

3. The head and facial region should generally be punctured superficially or obliquely, as the tissue and muscles are thin in those areas.

In order to avoid accidents, serious attention should be paid to the direction and depth of the insertion when puncturing the points of the ophthalmic region such as Bladder 1 (Jingming) and Stomach 1 (Chengqi), points on the neck such as Du 16 (Fengfu), Du 15 (Yamen) and Ren 22 (Tiantu), and points near the femoral artery or groin. These areas are particularly vulnerable to injury.

> HBV infection is usually preventable through a vaccine series. However, the only sure method of preventing HIV is abstinence from activities that involve the exchange of potentially infected body fluids.

## Dealing with Blood to Blood Contact

In the health care workplace, accidental contact with potentially contaminated blood or body fluids may be unavoidable. However, strict observance of standard universal precautions can prevent infection from exposure, especially from HBV, HCV and HIV.

---

48. 29 *CFR* 1910.1030 (d)(3)(ix)(A).

# Managing Used Instruments

*It is strongly recommended that used needles be isolated until they are sterilized or discarded.* Used needles present risk for practitioners, staff and children waiting for their parents. A sharps container for the used needles should be right beside the treatment table so that there is no delay in placing them away from potential accidental contact. Sharps containers should be red, of appropriate construction and labeled with the biohazard symbol.[49]

*It is strongly recommended that used-needle containers should be replaced regularly and not be over-filled above the fill mark or so that used needles are sticking out of the top. Replace a container when it is three-quarters full; do not attempt to push down the contents so that more may be placed inside.* This is critical for staff as well as practitioners, for studies document that a significant percentage of staff experience needlesticks while cleaning up sharps containers.[50]

If used needles are accidentally spilled, remember that they are contaminated and will in turn contaminate anything they touch. Use gloves and tweezers for picking them up and, if there is a possibility of dropping used needles on the practitioner's clothing and contaminating it, a gown or impervious apron should be used. Then the spill area should be cleaned with soap and water. Next all exposed surfaces should be wiped with a germicide since the HBV virus can survive on surfaces for more than one week at room temperature.[51] Bleach could also be used as the first-step cleanser, but since the contact with the contaminated surface deactivates the cleanser, the second cleaning with bleach must still be done. All materials used in the clean-up job should be discarded in double wrapping. The last step is handwashing. (The nuisance of cleaning up after a spill is a strong motivation for using containers that are stable and securely covered.)

If disposable needles are used, special containers are available for use as infectious waste receptacles to be disposed of through appropriate channels and according to local regulations. Any needles that are not in such specially designed containers must be sterilized before being discarded.

# Bleeding During Cupping

It is strongly recommended that if bleeding does occur during cupping, practitioners take the following steps:

1. *Gather gloves and cleaning materials,*
2. *Put on gloves,*
3. *Remove the cups, taking care to prevent body fluid from spreading or splashing,*
4. *Stop the bleeding through use of appropriate pressure,*
5. *Clean up any bleeding that has occurred,*

---

49. The Needlestick Safety Act requires that a log is kept next to the sharps container. In the event of a needlestick, the practitioner must document the type of date, type of needle and type of sharps container.

50. OSHA "Safe Needle Devices: Protecting Health Care Workers", October 1997.

51. CFR *op. cit.* 64012.

6. *Immediately isolate the cups,*
7. *Handle and dispose of all materials used in the cleaning process as biohazardous waste, and*
8. *Sterilize the cups using a double sterilization procedure.*

*It is recommended that chemical disinfectants be used on glass cups unless the manufacturer states that the cups may be autoclaved.* Since glass cups may crack during autoclaving, chemical sterilants should be used, according to manufacturer's direction, when bleeding has occurred.

*It is strongly recommended that disposable, plastic and rubber cupping devices that can not be sterilized be used on only one patient.* Cups with rubber or plastic parts may become damaged during autoclaving or when placed in a chemical sterilizing bath. Check with the manufacturer to determine if the cupping devices may be sterilized. If not, they should be used on only one patient. If bleeding occurs, the cups should be disposed of as biohazardous waste or sterilized in a chemical sterilant before disposal.

## Cleaning a Spill of Blood or Body Fluid

Cleaning accidental spills of blood or body fluid requires a two-step procedure similar to cleaning a spill of contaminated needles. Using rubber gloves, the spill should be cleaned once with soap and water. Then all exposed surfaces should be wiped with a germicide. Use a gown or impervious apron if there is a risk of contaminating your clothing during the clean up. Where there may be a risk of splashing or a very large spill, safety glasses and a disposable or sterilizable clothing protector should be worn. When disinfecting an extensive area with a hypochlorite (bleach) solution, disposable gloves may not be adequate, and may fail during the disinfecting process. Heavier gloves should be worn if this is a possibility. All materials used in the clean-up job should be discarded in double wrapping and hands should be washed at the end of the clean up.

### Laundering Sheets, Towels, Etc.

Cloth gowns, sheets, etc. are safe for reuse after ordinary laundering with hot water and soap or detergent. Chlorine bleach provides an extra margin of safety.[52]

## Disposing of Biohazardous Waste

When discussing biohazardous waste, the following terms are applicable:

*Biohazardous waste:* Any solid waste or liquid waste that may present a threat of infection to humans, including non-liquid human tissue and body parts, laboratory disease-causing agents, discarded sharps, human blood or clinic waste such as table paper or cotton balls that contain human blood, human blood products, and body fluids.

---

52. Favero, *op. cite* 18.

*Biohazardous waste generator:* A facility or person that produces or generates biohazardous waste including a wide range of facilities from hospitals to medical offices, from veterinary clinics to funeral homes. Licensed acupuncturists are included in this category.

OSHA has enacted specific rules concerning the handling and disposal of biohazardous or infectious waste in order to eliminate the exposure of employees, patients, and the public to disease-causing agents. These rules require:

❖ Waste generators must prepare, maintain, and implement a written plan to identify and handle such waste. They must also provide any employee that works in an area where biohazardous waste is kept an employee training program that explains procedures for on-site separation, handling, labeling, storage, and treatment of materials coming under this category.

❖ Biohazardous waste, except sharps (devices capable of puncturing, lacerating, or penetrating the skin), must be packaged in impermeable, red, polyethylene or polypropylene bags, and sealed. Discarded sharps must be separated from all other waste and placed in leak-resistant, rigid, puncture-resistant containers. All containers must be labeled properly, especially if the treatment and disposal is to take place off-site.

❖ In storing the packaged waste, care must be taken to place it in a designated area away from general traffic flow and accessible only to authorized personnel.

❖ Disposal methods include treatment by heat, incineration, steam sterilization, chemical treatment, or another equivalent method that renders the material inactive. State health departments are required to inspect all such waste generators to ensure compliance.

OSHA contains minimum standards established by the federal government. However, state and local regulations are permitted to be, and often are, more stringent, regarding the disposal of hazardous waste. These waste laws differ greatly from state to state and county to county. For example, some city, county or state governments require a permit and inspection for all offices that generate hazardous waste. Others require that used needles and other contaminated waste be picked up by a licensed contaminated disposal service. Still others require a permit to transport contaminated waste. It is important to be thoroughly familiar with the regulations in your locality. The state or county pollution control agency and/or health department is the best source for information and recommendations.

Whenever possible, it is advisable to have hazardous waste transported by an approved carrier. Should an individual, while transporting biohazardous waste, become involved in an accident, biohazardous materials may become strewn on a highway or other public space.

# WORKING IN PUBLIC HEALTH SETTINGS

There is a growing use of acupuncture in public health settings such as detox, AIDS, and TB clinics, as well as in institutions such as jails, public hospitals, community centers, and other social agencies that have group treatment rooms where several clients sit and receive ear or body acupuncture.

Clients may arrive together or separately, but usually do not have individual appointments. Many of these rooms do not have a sink in them. Some may have access to one nearby, but it is not always guaranteed.

Many of these settings aim at treating persons who are drug- and/or alcohol-addicted and who present with related and frequently multiple health and social problems such as TB, HIV infection, mental illness, homelessness, hunger or malnutrition, poverty, etc. These individuals frequently present with a long history of illness and a debilitated immune system.

The staff performing the acupuncture treatments are appropriately trained acupuncturists and/or acupuncture chemical dependency specialists, depending on state regulations. There are often other practitioners from different disciplines involved such as physicians, social workers, nurses, counselors, community workers, physician assistants, etc.

The characteristics of these clinics mandate some special discussion.

# Handwashing

Handwashing is one of the most problematic topics within a public health or group treatment setting. It is not realistic to expect that the practitioner will wash his or her hands in a sink after each treatment due to the volume of clients to be treated, the time and logistics that would be required, and frequently, the lack of facilities for handwashing *It is, however, strongly recommended that practitioners:*

➡ *Wash hands with soap and water before and after work shifts.*

➡ *Wash hands with soap and water, or if hand washing facilities are not in the immediate area, an alcohol-based or germicidal hand rub, immediately prior to performing any acupuncture.*

➡ *If no glove or finger cots are used, wash hands with soap and water between treatments as often as possible. An alcohol-based hand rub, prepackaged, disposable antiseptic towelette such as benzalkonium chloride (1:250) or a germicidal hand scrub should be used between treatments provided that only the needles, sterile packages and other materials needed for the treatment were touched. Practitioners may wish to carry a bottle of antiseptic handwash solution, readily available in most drug or grocery stores.*

➡ *Gloves should be available in the treatment area, and should be worn when there is a biohazardous spill such as significant bleeding from an auricular acupuncture point.*

➡ *Practitioners should wash their hands immediately with soap and water after critical instances such as contact with blood or a break in the clean field between or during treatments.*

# Choice of Instruments

State laws should be checked to determine if there are specific regulations regarding type of acupuncture needles to be used in public health settings. Disposable needles are recommended. Some states mandate that only disposable needles are used in chemical dependency treatments.

Guide tubes are not recommended for auricular acupuncture.

As always, care should be taken to monitor press needles for potential infections. This is particularly important in immuno-compromised patients.

## Positioning the Patient

When the patient is sitting up, it is important to make sure that, where possible, the patient has his or her head and neck supported, that the legs and arms are not crossed and that the person is comfortably seated.

Clients should be requested to use the bathroom prior to treatment. If a client does need to use the restroom during treatment, all needles should be removed and then replaced when he or she returns.

## Removing Needles

*When a practitioner is removing needles, it is critical to carry an impervious container so that the needles can be disposed of immediately.* In many public health settings it is important that needles be accounted for by counting the needles used. In settings such as jails the clients often may not leave until all needles are accounted for.

In some detox clinics clients remove their needles. In these instances the practitioner should always check for needles that may have dropped and for bleeding that may have occurred.

In all cases, practitioners should check chairs and surrounding areas for fallen needles before, during, and after each session, and after each client's needles are removed.

If needles fall out of the ear onto the clothing of the client during treatment, they should be removed with a minimum of disturbance.

Practitioners should instruct clients not to handle needles if the needles fall out or after removing them.

Delayed bleeding is common. Practitioners must be aware of this possibility. Patients should be monitored after needle removal and before leaving the premises.

## Managing Patient Accidents

If a client faints while sitting up, all needles should be removed immediately, legs raised to a horizontal position and the head lowered. It is also recommended that clients be placed safely on the floor if possible, making sure that the airways are not obstructed.

# CNT Outside the Office: Preparing and Using a Travel Kit

It is recognized that the travel-kit concept fills two important needs. One is that it helps develop sensitivity to the pitfalls of handling needles in a variety of settings. The second is that acupuncturists may be called on to travel, that is, to work outside the office. So the travel protocols have been retained as part of the CNT standards of practice.

Travel protocols include the details of preparation of the travel kit as well as treatment procedures that protect the sterility of the needles.

Preparing and using a travel kit embodies all the principles of clean needle technique and makes it feasible for the practitioner to observe responsible aseptic protocols in any setting. The design and contents of the kit, and procedures for its use, are given below.

## Travel Kit Contents

### Travel Kit Carrier

The travel kit should be carried in a briefcase or other appropriate hard-sided container or plastic case large enough to carry all the recommended equipment. It must have a tight closure. Plastic bags or soft-sided containers are not acceptable because they are not puncture-proof.

### Contents: Clean Items

1. Bags or containers to isolate equipment. Ziploc bags are commonly used in hospitals and are strongly recommended

2. Sealed and sterilized packages of needles. If guide tubes are used, a tube should be included in each needle packet when it is prepared for sterilization. If the sterile materials were sterilized by the practitioner, each packet should have an indicator of sterilization and should be marked with the date of sterilization.

3. Commercially prepared clean fields, clean paper, or any other surface such as a tray that will serve as a clean field packed in their own plastic bag or container.

4. Clean, dry cotton balls in their own plastic bag or container. Cotton balls need not be sterile.

5. Sterile gauze.

6. Rubber or vinyl gloves.

7. Antiseptic towelettes.

8. Tweezers or hemostat.

9. 70% isopropyl alcohol swabs.

**Medical Waste**

The final two items in the kit are packed in a shared ziplock bag. The purpose of this is to separate them from the clean equipment. This method of packing will clearly isolate the waste items from the clean materials.

1. The first item is a small paper bag (lunch bag size is adequate) with plastic liner to receive medical waste other than that which goes in the sharps container. An alternate to the plastic lined bag is a wax lined bag such as the type used to pack coffee. The purpose of the plastic or wax lining is to prevent absorption or leakage of wet material through the paper bag.

2. The second item is a *small commercial 'sharps' (bio-hazard) container.* The outside of the sharps container must remain clean as you will need to handle it. The sharps container should be carried in the sealable plastic bag that contains the lined waste bag. After use, it should be tightly closed and replaced in its designated bag, along with the folded waste bag. Do not place either of these items into the bag with the clean items. The bag that contains the sharps container and medical waste must be securely sealed before it is replaced into the hard-sided travel kit along with the clean bag.

## Preparing the Kit

The kit should be prepared in such a way that all items in it remain clean.

1. The hard-sided container must be washed in hot, soapy water and dried with a clean paper towel. Ziploc bags should be fresh from the package and free of rips and holes.

2. Hands should be washed before assembling the kit.

3. Paper toweling should be taken directly from its package and placed in a smaller plastic bag to ensure continued cleanliness.

4. Cotton balls should be taken directly from the stock bag and placed in a small plastic bag or other container. Clean hands or clean tongs should be the only things that have ever entered the stock bag.

5. Prepackaged alcohol swabs should be taken directly from their original box and placed in the kit. If they have been sitting open on a shelf the outer surfaces of the packets are no longer considered clean.

6. If disposable needles are used, they should be placed into the travel kit directly from the original box. If reusable needles are used, the needle packet should go directly from the sterilizer into the travel kit after it has dried.

## Treatment Protocol in a Travel Setting

1. Select an area to serve as the setting for the clean field. If necessary, clean it with soap and water and dry it thoroughly.

---

53. If a commercial sharps container is not used, the container should have a screw top, a wide base to prevent tipping and a wide-mouth to facilitate putting in the needles without touching the outside edges of the container.

2.  Wash hands for at least 10 seconds under running water, lathering well with soap. Liquid soap is recommended rather than bar soap, which may become contaminated. Special germicidal soap is needed if the practitioner has come into contact with blood or body fluids or if treating an immuno-compromised patient. If soap and water are unavailable, use an alcohol-based hand rub, antiseptic towelettes or an antiseptic scrub.

3.  Open the travel kit and remove the tray or towel that will serve as a clean field. Place it on the clean, dry work surface in a way that does not compromise the cleanliness of the surface that will serve as the clean field. For example, a clean folded towel should be handled by the four corners in order not to contaminate the center of the field. If alcohol is spilled or wet cotton is dropped on a previously clean field, it can no longer be considered clean since contaminants can wick into the field. A new clean field must be established before proceeding.

4.  Set out the materials from the travel kit. All clean items should be placed on the clean field, and should be handled so as to maintain their cleanliness. If something is dropped it cannot be picked up and placed in the clean field. It either must be discarded, or if cleanable, should be wiped clean with an alcohol swab. Open the alcohol swabs, cotton balls, etc., in such a way that the contents are accessible with a minimum of handling. The waste bag and the opened receptacle for contaminated needles should be placed **outside** the clean field.

5.  Needle packets may be opened and placed on your clean field right after you have set it up or they may be placed on the clean field and opened just prior to palpating and inserting the needle. When you do open a needle packet, your hands should be clean and you must handle the needles in a way that protects them from contact with anything that is not sterile. When the packet is opened, it should be folded back in such a way that when the needles are removed their shafts do not touch the part of the packet that was touched by the fingers while opening the packet.

6.  In the event the practitioner's hands become contaminated through contact with clothing or any other surface, a second hand cleansing would be necessary.

7.  Swab the points and allow the alcohol to dry.

8.  If a practitioner must place the needle inside a guidetube, the needle should be dropped into the tube, handle first, to minimize the risk of contaminating the point of the needle.

9.  Insert, manipulate, and withdraw the needle without touching the shaft of the needle at any time. If a guide tube is reused, it should be placed on the clean field between uses, since it has been handled and is no longer sterile.

10. If the practitioner wishes to 'close the hole', a clean, dry cotton ball should be used. The ball need not be sterile, but must be dry. A wet cotton ball or swab can wick up blood or other potential infectious material, bringing it into contact with the practitioner's fingers and increasing the risk of cross-infection.

11. Dispose of all cotton balls and alcohol swabs as they are used, placing them immediately in a plastic-lined paper bag carried for that purpose. They are not to be placed on the clean field after use and are not to be set down anywhere else but in the disposal bag. Close the disposal bag securely after the last used materials are placed inside.

12. Place the used needles in the sharps container. Close the lid securely.

13. Wash hands immediately after removing needles and before handling anything else.

14. Pack equipment correctly, placing the sharps container and waste in a separate bag.

15. Wash hands since the sharps container and waste bag were the last items handled.

CHAPTER 4

# Protocols for Sterilizing Instruments

MOST PRACTITIONERS TODAY USE prepackaged, presterilized disposable needles. However, use of disposable needles is only one aspect of maintaining sterility of needles and equipment. An understanding of sterilization is critical so practitioners may purchase appropriate equipment, inspect presterilized equipment to ensure that its sterility has not been compromised, store and handle it in a way that protects its sterilization and, if working in a clinic where acupuncture or plum blossom needles or cupping devices are reused, perform appropriate sterilization procedures. First, however, practitioners should check to ensure that the equipment is designed to be sterilized.

*It is strongly recommended that disposable equipment should not be reused or reprocessed without written approval from the manufacturer.*

## SUCCESSFUL STERILIZATION

Assurance of successful sterilization involves study and control of the complete process of sterilization. This process is outlined in the following sections:

1. Choosing the appropriate method and equipment.
2. Preparing and labeling instruments for sterilization.
3. Loading the sterilizer.

4. Monitoring that sterilization has occurred.
5. Ensuring proper function of the equipment.
6. Knowing what methods of sterilization are unacceptable.

## Choosing the Appropriate Sterilization Method and Equipment

In a clinical setting, sterilization by ethylene oxide, frequently used to sterilize prepackaged disposable equipment, is impractical. Therefore practitioners must look to other methods of sterilization for reusable equipment.

All acupuncture practitioners, even those who use sterilized disposable needles should know the sterilization process in case they work in a facility that:

• Does not use presterilized disposable acupuncture needles,

• Does not use presterilized disposable plum blossom needles,

• Uses cupping devices that require autoclaving.

Many experts consider the autoclave to be the method of choice for sterilization of acupuncture needles.[54] According to the CDCP, dry heat, ethylene oxide and chemical sporicides are also acceptable methods.[55] However, chemical sporicides are used primarily for first sterilization, disinfectants, antisepsis and non-autoclavable equipment. Boiling water does not sterilize, nor does soaking in alcohol.

### Autoclave

The autoclave delivers moist heat in the form of saturated steam under pressure. The sudden drop in pressure at the end of the cycle breaks down the cell walls of resistant spores and is an essential part of the sterilization process. If the autoclave does not vent and drop the pressure automatically, it must be done manually.

*It is critical that a pressurized steam bath, as provided by an autoclave, be maintained at 250 degrees Fahrenheit (121 degrees Centigrade), 15 pounds pressure for 30 minutes. The pressure must be released quickly at the end of the sterilization cycle*

Proper loading of the autoclave is essential. If materials are put in too densely the steam may not penetrate adequately. Packaging specially designed for autoclave should be used, since it will allow the steam to penetrate. Packages must be sealed and have space between them. Steel or glass containers must be vented during sterilization, in order for the steam to contact the needles. Lids must also be sterilized, but must not be placed on the containers until after the sterilization cycle is completed. Packets containing individual patients' needles must be sealed and labeled prior to sterilization.

---

54. APIC Guideline for Selection and Use of Disinfectants," *American Journal of Infection Control* 24, No. 4 (August 1996), pp. 313-342.

55. Current concern over sterilization is producing new technologies. These can most easily be judged by acceptability to the FDA. For example, gamma rays are used to sterilize some prepackaged disposable needles coming in from abroad. Since the FDA has approved them for import, the method of sterilization can be assumed to be acceptable.

The autoclave is designed to subject the equipment to a steam bath at high pressure. If the equipment is submerged in water being heated under pressure, sterilization is not accomplished. Residual air, which creates false readings on the gauges, is purged out of the autoclave to avoid interference with sterilization.

All autoclaved materials must be sterilized with autoclave tape and a label noting the date the material was autoclaved. Paper packets should be sealed with indicator tape if the packaging does not have imprinted indicators. Part of the tape will turn color after autoclaving, indicating that the package has been through the sterilizer. However, this is not an assurance that the contents are sterile. Should the tape not turn color, the materials must be considered to be nonsterile and be resterilized.

## Dry Heat Sterilization

Dry heat sterilizers provide heated air without steam pressure. Therefore they require longer sterilization time. Two hours of exposure to 338 degrees Fahrenheit is considered a safe time and temperature for dry heat sterilization. As with autoclave sterilization, it is important to space packages so that the dry hot air can have adequate contact with the instruments.

## Classification and Types of Chemical Disinfectants

Some instruments, such as those made of plastic can melt under the temperatures of either an autoclave or a dry heat sterilizer. To sterilize these, it is acceptable to use high level disinfectants. However, since disinfectants lose their strength by evaporation and with use, they must be used in the correct concentration and immersion time specified by the manufacturer and replaced appropriately. Since these chemicals may be destructive of the equipment being sterilized and it is difficult to rinse and package the equipment in a sterile manner, it is a better practice to purchase presterilized disposable equipment or equipment made of materials that can go through an autoclave or dry heat sterilizer. If disinfectants are used for sterilization, each item should be tested to determine if it can withstand the chemical sterilization before chemical sterilization is adopted as an office practice. Some disinfectants should be monitored for proper concentration and this monitoring should be documented. Check the manufacturer's specification for each disinfectant.

### Classifications of Disinfectants

Chemical germicides are classified by several different systems. The Environmental Protection Agency (EPA) classifies them according to claims by the manufacturer. It does not do independent tests of efficacy. Therefore, it is important to understand the labels to interpret the usefulness of a product for its purposes. Potential confusion in reading labels is shown in the comparison below between CDCP and EPA classifications.

"Sterilant" is the term used to describe a germicide that is used in such a way that it can actually sterilize. The same substance, called a sporicide by the EPA, might function as either a sterilant or a high-level disinfectant, depending on concentration, contact time, and temperature at which it is used.

The CDCP classification system uses the categories "high," "intermediate," and "low." The EPA classifications are "sporicides," "general disinfectants," "hospital disinfectants," and "sanitizers." "Sanitizers" correspond to the CDCP's "low-level disinfectants." Product labels often describe the level of germicidal action in terms of the infectious agents they challenge. The germicidal action could be high, intermediate, or low level, depending on the infectious agent that is challenged. Information on germicides is based on manufacturer's claims. Unfortunately, neither EPA nor FDA does testing to verify claims for level of germicidal action.

## Types of Disinfectants:

➡ Glutaraldehyde formulations have been found to be carcinogenic and are no longer recommended. Other sporocidal formulations are available.

➡ Dilutions of sodium hypochlorite (i.e., household bleach) solutions should be made within 24 hours of use. For smooth surfaces: 1:100 concentration. For porous surfaces or organic material: 1:10 concentration for 1 hour. (Note: Sodium hypochlorite is not recommended for acupuncture needles since if it is used for the recommended time and concentration, it will corrode needles and make them vulnerable to breakage after several applications.)

➡ Stabilized hydrogen peroxide in 6 to 25% concentrations is also capable of sterilization. Important: The hydrogen peroxide sold over the counter in pharmacies is 3% percent and is often old, resulting in effectiveness to less than a new 3% peroxide solution. Over the counter hydrogen peroxide solutions will not sterilize effectively. These substances are available under numerous brand names. It is essential to pay attention to the manufacturer's directions for use. The length of time required for these substances to act as sterilants may be destructive to the equipment being treated and reducing the time or concentration would defeat the intention of sterilization. It is therefore a good practice to purchase equipment made of materials that can go through the autoclave or dry heat sterilizer.

➡ Phenolic compounds such as Lysol cannot be used as sterilants, but are effective intermediate or low-level disinfectants for housekeeping purposes.

➡ Seventy-percent ethyl and isopropyl alcohol are classified as intermediate-level disinfectants. (Alcohol is also classified as an antiseptic for use on the skin.)

## Monitoring and Labeling of Disinfectants

The concentration of specific disinfectants can be monitored. This should be done if the manufacturer has the testing strips for monitoring. Monitoring increases the assurance that the solution is adequate for sterilization or high level disinfection.

OSHA regulations require that containers of disinfectant must be labeled if not in the original bottle. The label must include what the solution is, when it was mixed and its concentration.

The label must include what the solution is, when it was mixed and its concentration.

# THE DOUBLE STERILIZATION PROCEDURE

The proper sterilization of needles and other equipment is only one step in ensuring that the needle is sterile when it penetrates the skin. Equipment must also be prepared, cleaned, packaged and stored in such a way as to protect its sterility, and handled during treatment with attention to avoiding contamination.

Needles and other equipment that are reused must be cleaned. Cleaning is the physical removal of organic material. Cleaning itself will not kill infectious agents, but is a necessary step prior to sterilization because organic material such as blood or other body tissue may create a barrier that prevents disinfection or sterilization of the equipment.[56]

Since handling any used and therefore contaminated equipment in order to clean it creates risk of infection for the practitioner or staff, a basic protocol of double sterilization is recommended as follows.

## Preliminary Sterilization

For the protection of the practitioner and staff, used needles and other contaminated equipment should have a preliminary sterilization immediately after use. This should be done without cleaning or handling in any way.

*It is recommended that practitioners soak instruments in a chemical disinfectant for the preliminary sterilization.* Autoclaving does not sterilize the area under any blood or tissue that may remain on the equipment and may increase the difficulty in cleaning the items after the first sterilization. Use of a chemical disinfectant depends on several factors: selection of an appropriate disinfectant, proper concentration, and correct length of time.[57]

Chemical disinfectants vary a great deal by type and brand, so it is important to read labels and instructions carefully to determine whether, and under what conditions practitioners can obtain "sterilant" or "sporicide" action.

## Final Sterilization

*It is strongly recommended that reusable needles and other equipment be inspected carefully following the first sterilization.* This is to insure the absence of any damage or organic material remaining on the equipment after their first sterilization .

After the first sterilization it is safe to handle the instruments. Gloves should be worn during this procedure. The instruments should be soaked in water with or without detergent to loosen any material that may remain, wiped carefully and rinsed thoroughly. Each item should be washed separately. Determine if the needle is defective by a close visual inspection for creases in the shaft, corrosion, nicks, hooks at the tip of the shaft, dull points, etc. Draw the shaft of the needle through cotton

---

56. "APIC Guidelines" *op. cite.*

57. "APIC Guidelines" *op. cite.*

or across gauze to check for burrs. Use of electrical current through the needles may cause the needle shaft to pit or weaken with time. Check needles used with electrostimulation more often and more carefully. Discard defective needles in a sharps container. Those to be reused may then be sorted and packaged for final sterilization and storage as needed.

Chemical sterilants are not suitable for the second sterilization process. Whenever a disinfectant is used as a sterilant, it is essential that all traces of the chemical be washed off before using the instrument again. This would require the instruments to be handled with sterile gloves, washed in sterile water, and packaged in presterilized containers in order to protect sterility. These considerations do not present a problem for first-stage sterilization.

# Packaging and Labeling Instruments for Autoclave Sterilization

The following routine in-office procedures for packaging, labeling, loading and monitoring sterilization should be followed to ensure sterilization when using an autoclave.

## Packaging

Instruments should be packaged in the containers in which they will be stored and then sterilized again to destroy the contamination introduced by handling. There are many ways to package needles and other equipment safely for later use. Packaging must be judged by three criteria:

➡ Is it packaged in such a way that the steam or hot air has full access to each needle and other instrument during sterilization?

➡ Is all equipment fully protected from contamination once it is removed from the sterilizer?

➡ Can single needles be removed without contaminating the remaining ones?

*It is strongly recommended that all packaging for sterilized needles and other equipment provide protection from contamination during storage. Needles should be packaged in such a way to permit removal of single needles without contamination of the remaining ones.*

➡ Single-treatment packets: This is the safest system in this category. Enough needles for a treatment are inserted in the gauze in such a way that single needles can be removed one by one without touching the needles or the gauze with fingers. These gauze pads are then packaged individually in permeable paper wrapping designed for sterilization purposes. If guide tubes are used, one should be included in each packet.

➡ Covered trays: This system is less desirable since it is difficult to remove a needle without contaminating other needles. If this system is used, the needles should be placed obliquely or vertically in a bed of cotton or gauze, in a position that ensures that single needles can be removed without touching the shaft of a needle or the interior of the container. Sterile tweezers are best for this procedure because if a practitioner's fingers touch the shaft of a needle or the interior of the sterile tray the needles are contaminated. Since the handle of the tweezers becomes contaminated after use, the handle must not touch the sterile gauze.

When the tray is put into the sterilizer, the lid must also be placed in the sterilizer in such a way that the container is not sealed.

❖ When the sterilized material is dry, the container should be closed. The tray can then be removed from the sterilizer and carried to the treatment area or placed in storage.

*Cautions:* Sterilizing needles loose in the bottom of a tray is not desirable for two reasons. First, each time the tray is opened both the handles and the shafts of the needles are exposed to possible contaminants. Second, since it is difficult to remove a needle without touching the shaft of another, the needles *must* be removed with sterile tweezers in order to protect the sterility of the remaining needles. Between uses, the sterile tweezers may be stored in 70% isopropyl alcohol or between folds of sterile gauze as long as they have not been contaminated.

## Labeling Packages for Sterilization

*It is strongly recommended that all sterilized equipment be clearly marked so as to distinguish it from equipment that has not been sterilized.* The use of autoclave indicator tape on the exterior of the container is a suitable way to differentiate the sterile equipment if the packaging does not have imprinted indicators.

All individually sealed packages should be marked with the date of sterilization and load number. Any equipment in packages not used within an appropriate time must be resterilized before use. Any equipment in torn or opened packages, or sterile packages that ever become wet, must be resterilized before use.

# LOADING THE STERILIZER

*It is critical that the sterilizer be loaded with enough air space between packages to permit full circulation and penetration of steam or hot air.* If more than one layer is placed on a shelf, packages should be spaced and criss-crossed to allow for circulation. All impervious containers must be uncovered during sterilization. Steam or hot air cannot penetrate to instruments in a sealed container. Packaging materials must be designed for the particular type of sterilizer being used.[58]

# MONITORING THAT STERILIZATION HAS OCCURRED

Monitoring sterilization means checking regularly to see that the equipment being run through the

---

58. CDCP, "Infection Control In Dentistry: Bloodborne Disease Transmission", *Promotion: Division of Oral Health,* July 3, 2000

sterilizer has actually been rendered sterile. This is accomplished by including biological monitors such as spore ampules or spore strips in the load. *It is strongly recommended that biological indicators be used after any repair has been done on the sterilizer and once a week or according to manufacturer's instructions to verify that the sterilizer is functioning properly.*

Indicator strips that change color are not a reliable indication that sterilization has taken place. The color changes are gradual as the temperature increases but do not indicate how long the highest temperature was maintained. Therefore the strips do not provide assurance that the appropriate temperature has been reached and maintained for the necessary length of time. Similarly, glass-enclosed melting pellet indicators show that a specified temperature has been reached, but do not indicate how long that temperature was maintained. Nor do they indicate whether steam has penetrated appropriately or whether the pressure has been released rapidly. Biological indicators should therefore be used once a week or according to manufacturer's directions to assure proper equipment functioning. Indicator strips placed on the outside of packages before being processed are useful to identify containers of equipment that have been through the sterilizer but are not reliable.

Biological indicators are available for use in autoclaves and in dry heat sterilizers. These indicators are packets containing highly resistant bacteria spores that are placed in a normal load, buried in the center of the load to mimic the longest distance the steam must travel to get to the materials in the center of the load. The packets are then incubated under appropriate conditions. If there is any bacterial growth, the packet indicates that the sterilization cycle failed; that either the time or the temperature was inadequate.

Rapid-read biological indicators are available that can be processed onsite. These are small ampules that are easier to handle than the packages. Check with the manufacturer of the sterilizer or a medical supply company to obtain the rapid read biological indicators.

The Centers for Disease Control has advised the dental profession to run a biological indicator once a week.[59] Some states have their own requirement regarding frequency of monitoring. Check with the appropriate state regulatory body for current requirements. The results of the monitoring process should be maintained in a sterilization log, which is usually kept with the sterilizer.

*It is strongly recommended that load logs be maintained for each load that is run in the sterilizer.* This log should include a load number, the items included in the load, the date, the results of the indicator paper and the result of the biological indicator (if one was run), the temperature, length of processing and if the pressure was attained. The person running the load should initial the log each time a load has been entered. This improves tracking so that it is easier to identify which patient's needles were processed in what load.

It is strongly recommended that there be a written procedure for when the biological indicator is positive. This would include tracking and recall of equipment that was processed in the load that failed as well as follow-up of the patients that may have been exposed to the questionably contaminated items.

## Ensuring Proper Functioning of Equipment

There are several ways in which the sterilization process can break down. Mechanical fault or procedural error could invalidate the whole sterilization process and leave practitioners, patients, and office staff at risk of infection. Equipment failure is a continuing risk in sterilization. Seals can leak and gauges and timers can become inaccurate. In addition, human error is always a possibility even with equipment that has not become faulty.

All equipment should be operated, cleaned and serviced regularly according to the recommendations of the manufacturer. Otherwise sterilization may not be achieved. Autoclaves need to have valves, seals, and timers checked. Dry heat sterilizers should be checked with a separate internal thermometer to verify the accuracy of the gauge built into the equipment.

A record of all autoclave maintenance and testing must be kept, including routine testing and maintenance, and repairs. A certified sterilizer technician familiar with the model being used must perform all repairs. Any sign that the autoclave is not performing as required must result in the immediate cessation of the use of the autoclave until the problem is solved.

Biological monitors should be used before using new equipment, after any repair has been done on the sterilizer and as directed by the manufacturer or once a week thereafter. Careful records should be kept of the date and outcome of each inspection, servicing, and monitoring procedure. This is important both for office management purposes and for use in any possible legal actions involving cross-infection.

In addition to a biological indicator, an indicator paper or packet should be run at least weekly to determine if steam is reaching all areas of the sterilizer and if the vacuum is successfully removing all of the steam. Check with the manufacturer of the sterilizer or a medical supply company for appropriate monitoring equipment.

The failure to perform any of the above steps or complete the manufacturer's maintenance and validation procedures could result in a failure of sterilization, leading to the use of nonsterile instruments that were believed to be sterile.

# UNACCEPTABLE PROCEDURES FOR STERILIZATION

## Boiling Water

The use of the word sterilization is incorrect when applied to boiling water. Several investigators have shown that neither boiling water (212 °F or 100°C) nor flowing (non-pressurized) steam heat are adequate for the destruction of resistant bacterial spores and some viruses.

## Alcohol

Alcohol is NOT an effective sterilizing agent and should not be used for the purpose of sterilization. This is not to suggest that alcohol is inadequate for other important functions in an acupuncture clinic. It is the substance of choice for cleaning the skin.

## Pressure Cookers

Pressure cookers are not designed with sufficient accuracy of temperature, heat and pressure to ensure sterilization. They also do not have automatic evacuation of air and are not designed to prevent the acupuncture equipment from being submerged in the water. Thus they are not acceptable for sterilization in a health care setting.

# SUMMARY OF STERILIZATION EQUIPMENT AND PROCEDURES

➡ All instruments that penetrate the skin must be sterile.

➡ Acceptable sterilization modes convenient for the average clinic include:

❖ *Autoclave:* 30 minutes at 250 degrees F. (121 degrees Centigrade), 15 pounds pressure with rapid decompression at the end of the cycle.

❖ *Dry Heat*: two hours at 338 degrees F.

❖ *Chemical sporicidal sterilant:* according to manufacturer's instructions, for first sterilization only.

➡ Biological monitoring is the most reliable assurance that the sterilizer is functioning properly.

➡ All sterilizers should be checked for mechanical function periodically, according to manufacturer's instructions.

➡ The loading of the sterilizer must be done in such a way that steam or dry heat can penetrate every container or package.

➡ Double sterilization is recommended to protect practitioner and staff from the risk of cross-infection.

❖ Preliminary sterilization in a chemical disinfectant takes place without any handling by bare hands of equipment that has become contaminated, such as needles after they are withdrawn from the patient or cups or plum blossom needles that have been contaminated by blood.

❖ Soak needles and other equipment in water, with or without detergent, to loosen any material on the equipment.

❖ Using gloves, wipe carefully and rinse thoroughly.

❖ Check needles and other equipment for pitting, burrs, cracking, corrosion or other signs of wear.

❖ Repackage for resterilization in packaging designed to protect needles and other equipment from contamination during storage and use. Label with date and load number.

❖ Second sterilization.

➡ The sterilized equipment should then be handled and stored properly.

➡ The storage area should be maintained in a clean and dry manner and should be cleaned on a routine basis.

CHAPTER **5**

# Risk Reduction

R ISK REDUCTION IS A TERM that is used to describe procedures and techniques that will reduce practitioners' vulnerability to lawsuit or legal sanctions. Use of CNT and universal precautions with every patient are forms of risk reduction. However, in addition to complying with the specific requirements of acupuncture and Oriental medicine practice acts, practitioners must comply with state and federal statutes regarding general medical practice such as informed consent, recordkeeping, patient confidentiality, reporting of communicable disease and maintenance of an Exposure Control Plan.

Although in many instances acupuncturists are not specifically mentioned in the relevant state statutes, it is recommended that practitioners be aware of and comply with the state law pertaining to informed consent, recordkeeping and patient confidentiality. Not only is there an ethical principle that practitioners should practice in accordance with these general medical guidelines, not to do so may cause practitioners to be vulnerable to civil and criminal penalties.

Practitioners should become acquainted with their state's regulations. Usually these laws may be found in the state public health code or health and safety code rather than the acupuncture practice act. An introduction to the issues is presented below. However, practitioners should contact their state board or local health department for further information.

## OFFICE ENVIRONMENT

Acupuncturists must conduct their practice in such a way as to ensure, so far as is reasonably practicable, that persons who may be affected thereby are not exposed to risks to their health or safety. This duty extends to both patients and employees. It is by following recognized standards established by OSHA that this duty can be fulfilled. In connection with safety aspects, particular attention is drawn to the following:

1. All floors, passages, and stairs shall be of sound construction and properly maintained and should be kept free from obstruction and from any substance likely to cause persons to slip.

2. A substantial handrail and adequate lighting should be provided for every staircase.

3. Adequate lighting must be provided and maintained in all office spaces.

4. All equipment should be subjected to regular inspection and preventative maintenance.

5. All electrical installations should be in accordance with local codes.

6. Every chair, seat, or couch in the premises should be kept clean, and maintained in proper repair.

7. Floors should be easily cleaned. Carpeting in areas where biohazardous waste is generated or stored is not recommended since it is difficult to clean up spilled needles or fluids.

Practitioners should also consult OSHA requirements, Section 3 for provisions regarding maintenance and use of work areas, signs, etc.

# Informed Consent

It is generally recognized that the relationship between a physician and his or her patient comes into being because of the patient's need, and trust in the skill, learning, and experience of the physician. The physician may not, under ordinary circumstances, impose services upon another without that person's consent.

Consent is authorization by the patient or a person authorized by law to consent on the patient's behalf. This authorization changes a treatment from nonconsensual to consensual. Although most consent cases involve physicians, the principles of law concerning the nature of consent are equally applicable to acupuncturists.

An acupuncturist may be held liable for malpractice if, in rendering treatment to a patient, he or she does not make a proper disclosure to the patient of the risks involved in the procedure.

Written consent provides visible proof of consent. A valid, written consent must include the following elements:

❖ It must be signed.
❖ It must show that the procedure was the one consented to.
❖ It must show that the person consenting understood the nature of the procedure, alternatives, the risks involved, and the probable consequences.
❖ The patient should fill in the date of signing.

Oral consent, if proven, is just as binding as written consent. However, oral consent may be difficult to prove in court.

Informed consent is particularly important when using techniques that might be interpreted as causing damage to the body, such as direct moxibustion and cupping or gua sha, which may leave bruises.

# Maintaining Accurate Patient Records

Records should be kept of all patient visits and treatments performed. The medical record should be a complete, accurate, up-to-date report of the medical history, condition, and treatment of each patient. *It is recommended that acupuncturists follow standard medical charting procedures such as the SOAP notes:*

❖ *Subjective (information reported by the patient),*

❖ *Objective (information gathered by the practitioner, i.e., tongue, pulse, palpation, etc.),*

❖ *Assessment (of the patient's condition and treatment progress) and*

❖ *Plan (treatment record for the day, including points, herbs, dietary and lifestyle recommendations, new diagnosis, referral (if any), etc.)*

*Daily treatment records should include the points and treatment procedures for each visit, for example,' moxa on St 36' or 'electrical stimulation UB 18 and 23 (bilateral)'.*

Treatment records are maintained primarily to provide accurate and complete information about the care and treatment of patients. They are the principal means of communication between health practitioners in matters relating to patient care and serve as a basis for planning the course of treatment. They are also the practitioner's record of what occurred if there is a complaint or law suit. Legislation and regulations concerning medical records vary from state to state. Many states require medical records to be kept for a specific length of time after treatment. Some states detail the information required concerning the patient's treatment. Others simply declare that the medical record should be adequate, accurate, or complete.

## DAILY APPOINTMENT SCHEDULES

Records of daily appointment schedules must be retained. In an investigation of an outbreak of HBV particularly, nothing is more important than that an accurate record has been kept of names and addresses of all patients and dates of treatments. Since hepatitis B has a long and varied incubation period, lack of recorded information about patients' treatment at relevant times may prevent the proper investigation of any cross-infection related to HBV.

## PATIENT CONFIDENTIALITY

Practitioners should be aware that as a general rule practitioners may not release information regarding a patient, either verbally or in writing, without the patient's consent. Practitioners may, however, discuss cases with other health care professionals so long as there is no identifying information provided.

Both federal and state confidentiality laws govern the release of information relative to HIV, substance abuse or substance abuse treatment, sexually transmitted diseases, mental health and other medical conditions. Disclosure without the patient's consent may make a practitioner vulnerable to criminal prosecution or a civil law suit.

# Reporting of Communicable Disease and Abuse

State laws vary with regard to requirements for medical practitioners to report known or suspected communicable diseases, child or elder abuse.

# OSHA exposure control plan

Employers of health care workers are encouraged to participate in the task of controlling the spread of blood-borne pathogens such as HBV/HIV by disseminating preventive information in the workplace through a detailed exposure control plan (ECP). Each employer having an employee(s) with occupational exposure must develop such a plan designed to eliminate or minimize employee exposure incidence. Practitioners who have employees, whether they be a receptionist or a janitor, who may be exposed to blood borne pathogens by pulling needles, emptying the trash, assisting patients in dressing and undressing, should have an ECP. Practitioners who share office space with other practitioners, including treatment room or storage area for biohazardous waste, must also develop an ECP.

The ECP should include the following exposure determination criteria:

1. A list of job classifications where all employees have occupational exposure,

2. A list of job classifications where some employees have occupational exposure, and

3. A list of all tasks and procedures (or closely related groups of activities) in which occupational exposure occurs.

The ECP should also provide a schedule and methods of implementation of precaution procedures, and procedures for evaluating exposure incidents. A copy of the plan must be made available to all employees. The plan must be reviewed and updated annually, or whenever new or revised tasks or procedures are added to the practice, or if new positions are created that may have exposure potential.

OSHA requires that the ECP contain at least the following components:

**Methods of Compliance**

1. Engineering and Work Practice Controls: Includes requirements for handwashing facilities, sharps containment, maintenance and use of work areas, procedures involving blood or potentially infectious materials, and handling of equipment that may become contaminated.

2. Personal Protective Equipment: Covers the provision and use of items such as gloves, gowns, masks, and other pieces of clothing or equipment when occupational exposure is possible. Latex-free gloves must be provided if an employee is allergic to latex

3.  Housekeeping: Includes requirements for maintaining the worksite in a clean and sanitary condition, sharps containment and disposal, disposal of contaminated waste, and handling of contaminated laundry.

### Communication With Employees

1.  Labels and Signs: Includes requirements for BIOHAZARD labels and warning signs, containers, and bags.
2.  Information and Education/Training: New employees must be offered a hepatitis B vaccine and receive bloodborne pathogen education prior to having contact with blood or body fluids.

### Record Keeping for the Exposure Control Plan

1.  Medical Records: Covers data required for employee medical records and confidentiality availability controls.
2.  Training Records: Covers data required for employee training records and file maintenance requirements

Practitioners should contact their local health department or hospital to obtain further information regarding OSHA training.

# SUMMARY OF UNIVERSAL PRECAUTIONS

The Centers for Disease Control and Prevention have developed procedures to help health care workers protect themselves from a variety of possible infections, including HBV and HIV. In general, these precautions include the use of an appropriate barrier (gloves, gowns, masks, goggles, etc.) to prevent contact with infected body fluids. Additionally, standard sterilization and disinfection measures as well as infectious waste disposal procedures must be followed.

These practices are especially important for all health care professionals who participate in invasive procedures. In addition to gowns, gloves, and surgical masks, protective eyewear or face shields should be worn where generation of droplets or splashing of body fluids is possible. If the protective barrier becomes torn, it should be replaced immediately or as soon as patient safety permits. In the event of injury to the health care practitioner, the barrier should be removed and the wound treated promptly. Any such injury should also be followed up with an incident report.

Since medical history and examination cannot reliably identify all patients infected with HBV/HIV or other bloodborne pathogens, infection prevention methods should be used consistently for ***all*** patients.

### Summary of CDCP's Universal Precaution Recommendations [60]

❖ All health care workers (HCWs) should adhere to universal precautions, including the appropriate use of hand washing, protective barriers, and care in the use and disposal of needles and other sharp instruments.

---

60.  Revised and updated July 30,1999.

❖ Hands should be washed before and after patient contact, and immediately if hands become contaminated with blood or other body fluids. Hands should also be washed after removing gloves.

❖ HCWs should comply with current guidelines for disinfection and sterilization of reusable devices used in invasive procedures.

❖ Instruments and other reusable equipment used in performing invasive procedures should be appropriately disinfected and sterilized as follows:

— Equipment and devices that enter the patient's vascular system or other normally sterile areas of the body should be sterilized before being used for each patient.

— Equipment and devices that touch intact mucous membranes, but do not penetrate the patient's body surfaces, should be sterilized when possible and should undergo high-level disinfection if they cannot be sterilized before being used for each patient.

— Equipment and devices that do not touch the patient or that only touch intact skin of the patient need only be cleaned with a detergent or as indicated by the manufacturer.

❖ Gloves should be worn whenever there is a possibility of contact with body fluids.

❖ Body fluids to which universal precautions apply: blood, serum/plasma, semen, vaginal secretions, cerebrospinal fluid, vitreous fluid, synovial fluid, pleural fluid, pericardial fluid, peritoneal fluid, amniotic fluid, and wound exudates.

❖ Body fluids when blood is visible: sweat, tears, sputum, saliva, nasal secretions, feces, urine, vomit, breast milk.

❖ HCWs who have exudative lesions or weeping dermatitis should refrain from all direct patient care and from handling patient-care equipment and devices used in performing invasive procedures.

❖ Sharp objects represent the greatest risk for exposures. Contaminated needles should never be bent, clipped, or recapped. Immediately after use, contaminated sharp objects should be discarded into a puncture-resistant biohazard container designed for this purpose. Needle containers should never be overfilled; containers should be sealed and discarded when two-thirds to three-quarters full.

❖ Contaminated equipment that is reusable should be cleaned of visible organic material, placed in an impervious container, and placed in a designated place for decontamination and reprocessing.

❖ Masks should be worn whenever there is a possibility of splashing or splattering of body fluids or with an active TB patient.

❖ Gowns should be worn if possible contamination of exposed skin or clothing is likely.

❖ Spills of blood or blood-containing body fluids should be cleaned up using a solution of household bleach (sodium hypochlorite) and water in a 1:100 solution for smooth surfaces and 1:10 for porous surfaces. Diluted bleach solutions should be no more than 24 hours old.

❖ Current data indicate that HCWs infected with HIV or HBV who perform invasive procedures that are not exposure-prone, pose no risk provided they practice the recommended surgical or dental techniques and observe universal precautions, and follow recommendations for sterilization and disinfection.

❖ Medical/surgical/dental organizations and institutions at which these procedures are performed should identify exposure-prone procedures.

❖ To minimize the risks for exchange of body fluids during resuscitation procedures, pocket masks or mechanical ventilation devices should be readily available where these procedures are likely to be needed.

CHAPTER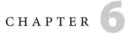

# What to do for: Accidents, etc.

THE FOLLOWING PAGES LIST the most important safety concerns in the practice of acupuncture. In some areas there are specific recommendations. In other areas there are no recommendations and the discussion is rather brief. Please refer to current texts for information on safe practice.

## ACCIDENTS

Although studies show that acupuncture accidents seldom occur if the practitioners are well trained,[61] precautions must be taken to prevent them. If an accident does occur, either due to needling that causes trauma or injury, or due to another accident or injury while the patient is in the practitioner's office and under his/her care, the practitioner should be prepared to evaluate the situation and respond quickly.

It is suggested that practitioners have a list of emergency numbers readily available. Include the local number for emergency medical assistance, hospitals, fire, police, and the numbers of professionals available for advice, consultation, or referral.

---

61. National Acupuncture Foundation, *Safety Record of Acupuncture* (2002).

# NEEDLESTICKS

One of the most common forms of cross-infection is needlesticks. In fact, studies show that 58% to 80% of the exposures to HIV within a health care setting are through needlesticks.[62]

Risk of infection from needlesticks involving an infected patient is 6% to 30% for HBV[63] and 0.5% for HIV.[64] These figures emphasize the need for practitioners and staff to handle contaminated needles properly as well as the need for an Exposure Control Plan, as stipulated by OSHA, which mandates that employers establish exposure control plans that include post-exposure follow-up for their employees and to comply with incident reporting requirement.[65, 66]

*In the event that a practitioner or staff member sticks him or herself with a contaminated needle, it is strongly recommended that he or she consult a physician immediately and follow the office exposure control plan.* (A contaminated needle is any needle that has been through a patient's skin and has not yet been sterilized.)[67]

Once an exposure has occurred, the individual should follow the process outlined in the exposure control plan. Local laws regarding consent for testing source individuals should be followed. Policies should be in place for testing source individuals in situations where consent cannot be obtained. Testing of the source individual should be done at a location where appropriate pre-test counseling is available; post-test counseling and referral for treatment should be provided.

CDC recommends testing the source (patient) and the person exposed for diseases or immunity to the following diseases: hepatitis B, hepatitis C, and the presence of the AIDS virus. The source should be tested as soon as possible. Based on the type and amount of exposure and if the source tests positive for HIV, the employee should be offered post-exposure prophylaxis for HIV. This testing should ideally be done within 2 hours of the exposure and the treatment should start as soon as possible, if required.

The source should be tested for hepatitis B surface antigen, hepatitis C antibody, and HIV. The person exposed should be tested for hepatitis B surface antibody, hepatitis C antibody and HIV. The exposed person is tested for hepatitis C and HIV to determine at the time of exposure whether the person had the disease.

---

62. OSHA "Safe Needle Devices" *op cite.*

63. James Hersey and Linda Martin, *op. cit.* 244.

64. OSHA "Safe Needle Devices" *op cite.*

65. "Updated U.S. Public Health Service Guidelines for the Management of Occupational Exposures to HBV, HCV and HIV and Recommendations for Postexposure Prophylaxis", MMWR, 6/29/01/50(RR/1); pp. 1-42.

66. Congress enacted new provisions, effective April 18, 2001, that require employers to maintain a log of injuries from contaminated sharps, noting the type of sharps and sharps container, next to each sharps container.

67. For current needlestick recommendations, contact the National Clinicians' Post-Exposure Prophylaxis Hotline at 1-888-448-4911

Additional follow-up testing is also recommended.[68]

*It is recommended that practitioners consult with an infectious disease physician to obtain the most current recommendations for treatment.*

Due to the risk of needlestick, the CDCP strongly recommends immunization against HBV for HCWs. OSHA requires that HBV vaccine must be made available to all employees who have occupational exposure. The vaccine must be provided without cost to the employee and in a convenient location. Any employee who does not want the vaccine must sign a statement declining the vaccine. Options should be discussed with a physician before making a decision.

OSHA also requires that employers maintain confidential medical records on all employees including information about the employees' hepatitis B vaccination status and a medical evaluation of an employee after an exposure incident. The records must be retained for at least the duration of the employment plus 30 years.

# Pain or Trauma on or After Insertion

Needle insertion should not elicit an unnecessarily painful response in the vast majority of patients. Avoid unnecessary pain as the needle pierces the skin by careful and considerate insertion. If patients consistently or often feel pain on insertion, the practitioner's technique must be re-evaluated and improved. Defective, dull, or needle gauges inappropriate to the point being needled may also cause undue pain.

Pain occurring when the needle enters deep into tissue may be due to the needle striking an artery wall, periosteum, tendon, or nerve. Appropriate measures should be taken, such as lifting the needle until it is just beneath the skin, changing the direction, and inserting it again carefully.

Pain occurring when the needle is rotating in a wide arc is generally because the shaft of the needle is entwined with fibrous tissue. Various methods may be taken to relieve the pain such as gently rotating the needle back and forth until the fiber is released.

# Fainting

*Symptoms:* During acupuncture treatment, symptoms such as dizziness and vertigo, oppressive feeling in the chest, palpitation, nausea, and pallor may occur. In severe cases, there may be such signs as cold extremities, cold sweating, weak pulse, loss of consciousness, hypotension, and shock.

---

68. For the complete guide, *Public Health Service Guideline for the Management of Health-Care Workers Exposures to HIV and Recommendations for Post-exposure Prophylaxis,* see CDC's web address: http://www.cdc.gov/mmwr/preview/mmwrhmtl/000053722.

*Cause:* Nervous tension, hunger, fatigue, extreme weakness of the patient, or overly forceful manipulation resulting in excessive stimulation.

*Management:* The needle should be removed immediately and the patient allowed to lie flat with the feet or legs slightly elevated. The practitioner may offer the patient warm drinks or administer acupuncture treatment according to training. Generally, allow the patient to recover on his or her own unless unusual signs of distress are evident, such as difficulty in breathing.

Two common acupuncture techniques for relief of faintness or actual resuscitation are:

1.  Press point GV 26 (Renzhong) with the fingernail, or puncture GV 26 and Pericardium 6 (Neiguan);

2.  Press, moxa, or needle Stomach 36 (Zusanli) if needling has been done in the upper half of the body, and L.I. 4 (Hegu) if needling had been done in the lower part of the body.

Generally the patient will respond to these measures, but if the symptoms are still unrelieved, call for emergency medical assistance.

*Prevention:* It is advisable to treat patients lying down if they are weak, tired, fasting, or in a nervous state. Needle manipulation on these patients should be gentle, and the facial expression and color of the patients must be observed at all times in order to detect reactions as early as possible and prevent accidents. If patients are sitting up for treatment, make sure they are well supported.

# STUCK NEEDLE

After the needle is inserted, it may be difficult or impossible to rotate, lift and thrust, or withdraw. The cause is usually due to spasm of the muscle or overly wide amplitude of rotation of the needle, leading to fibrous tissue becoming tangled around the shaft of the needle.

To manage this, reassure the patient if she is nervous, ask her to relax her muscles, then massage or tap the skin around the point, after which the needle should be easily removable. If the needle is still held fast, ask the patient to lie calmly for a while or give another puncture nearby so as to relax the muscle. If the needle is still entangled in fibrous tissue, turn it slightly in the opposite direction until it becomes loose, then withdraw it.

# BROKEN NEEDLE

A broken needle may occur if there are cracks or erosions of the shaft of the needle, especially at the junction with the handle, if the quality of the needle is poor, if the patient has changed position to too great an extent, if there is a strong spasm of the muscle, if excessive force is used in manipulating, if the needle has been struck by an external force, or if a bent needle has been rigidly withdrawn.

To manage a broken needle the acupuncturist should remain calm and advise the patient not to move so as to avoid causing the broken part of the needle to sink deeper. If a part of the needle is still exposed above the skin, remove with forceps. If it is on the same level with the skin, press the tissues around the site gently until the broken end is exposed, then take it out with forceps. If it is completely under the skin, seek medical help immediately. Do not cut the flesh to get access to the needle.

In order to prevent broken needles, the needles should be carefully inspected prior to treatment. The necessity of remaining still while undergoing therapy should be explained to the patient. When manipulating the needle, be sure not to use too great a force, and when the needle is retained in place, the shaft of the needle should remain exposed above the skin.

*It is strongly recommended that a needle never be inserted up to the handle.*

# ACCIDENTAL INJURY TO ORGAN(S)

If an important organ is accidentally injured during acupuncture treatment, the acupuncturist must take emergency measures at once. The following are the circumstances that may occur and measures to be taken:

*Lung:* If the needle is thrust too deeply or in an incorrect direction into the points of the chest, back or supraclavicular fossa, traumatic pneumothorax may result. Clinical symptoms are pain in the chest and cough. In severe cases there may be dyspnea, pallor, cyanosis, coma, etc. Fatality may occur in very severe cases or if the case is not managed properly.

*It is strongly recommended that if a pneumothorax is suspected that the following actions be taken:*

1. *Carefully withdraw the needle immediately. The worst damage is tearing of tissue caused by breathing or coughing with the needle still in.*

2. *Encourage the patient to lie calmly.*

3. *The patient should be taken to the hospital; if the symptoms are severe, call for emergency help.*

*Heart, liver, spleen, and kidney:* Prior to acupuncture, special care should be taken to examine the patient for any suspected organ enlargement. Abnormal changes in the internal organs may come from diseases such as cardiac disease, hepatomegaly, or splenomegaly.

Puncturing the liver or spleen may cause a rupture with bleeding. Symptoms are abdominal pain, rigidity of the abdominal muscles, and/or rebound pain upon pressure. Puncturing the kidney may cause pain in the lumbar region, tenderness and pain upon percussion around the kidney region, and bloody urine. Coma may result if blood loss is great.

*It is strongly recommended that if there are signs that an organ may have been punctured that the patient be taken to the hospital or emergency medical help be called.*

*Brain and spinal cord:* If the needle enters too deeply, or if there is inappropriate manipulation in such points as GV 15 (Yamen) or GV 16 (Fengfu), there may be bleeding and other severe consequences. Clinical manifestations are convulsions, paralysis, and coma.

*It is strongly recommended that if any of the above symptoms occurs emergency medical help be called for immediately.*

*Blood vessels:* When giving acupuncture treatment, one should avoid puncturing large blood vessels. Local bleeding may occur, especially in old people who have little elasticity of their blood vessels. If this happens, measures should be taken to stop bleeding and to help absorption. For a vein, direct pressure for 30 seconds to 1 minute should be sufficient; for an artery, up to five minutes of direct pressure may be required.

*Other organs:* Special care should also be taken when puncturing in regions close to the stomach, intestine, urinary bladder, gallbladder, and eyes.

## HIGH-RISK PATIENTS

Under universal precautions, all patients should be treated the same.

CHAPTER 7

# Safety Issues when Using Special Techniques

## ELECTRICAL STIMULATION

*It is strongly recommended that electrical stimulation not be used on any part of the body of patients with pacemakers or other electronic implants.* Also, some patients with a history of seizure disorders may not respond well to electrical stimulation.

*It is strongly recommended that since electrical stimulation may interfere with the action of the heart muscle, electrical stimulation not be applied from one side of the chest across to the other side of the chest (front to back or side to side) in the region of the heart.*

In regard to the amount of stimulation, the level of stimulus should never approach the sensation of pain.

Certain type of metals should be avoided for use in electroacupuncture such as silver needles, which are softer than stainless steel, for they may electrolyze in the body very quickly and may result in a toxic reaction. Stainless steel needles are safe to use with electrical stimulation, but it is advisable to use relatively thick needles, such as Chinese 32 gauge or Japanese #5, to minimize risk of breakage.

# MOXIBUSTION

Practitioners should avoid causing burns and be aware that each person has a different tolerance to heat. It is important to be especially careful of persons who have conditions where sensitivity of local nerves may be diminished, such as in neural injury, diabetes, or pathology resulting in paralysis, because they are especially susceptible to burns. Even chemical heat devices such as "Hot Spots" and heat lamps have been known to burn diabetics.

When using indirect moxa on the needle be sure to protect the patient's skin from any falling moxa or ashes. If using direct moxa, it is suggested that the practitioner fully explains the technique to the patient and asks the patient to sign an informed, written consent form prior to using the technique of direct moxa.

If a patient has been burned, infection is the primary concern. If the burn is very small in area, and first or second degree, apply sterile gauze over a burn ointment. If a burn is severe, or if there are any signs of infection, refer the patient to a physician.

# BLEEDING TECHNIQUES

When the practitioner bleeds an acupuncture point using a lancet or acupuncture needle, it is suggested that two layers of gloves be used. This allows the practitioner to remove a glove and reglove if the glove becomes bloody during the procedure, without concern about direct contact with blood.

APPENDIX **1**

# Where to Find More Information

CDC National AIDS Hotline:

    (English) 24 hours a day, 7 days a week. . . . . . . . . . . . . . . . . . . . . . . . . . . . . . . . . . 1-800-342-AIDS

    (Spanish) 7 days a week, 8:00 a.m. - 2:00 a.m. EST . . . . . . . . . . . . . . . . . . . . . . 1-800-344-SIDA

    (TTD/TTY for deaf and hearing impaired) . . . . . . . . . . . . . . . . . . . . . . . . . . . . 1-800-243-7889

CDC National Prevention Information Network . . . . . . . . . . . . . . . . . . . . . . . . . . 1-800-458-5231

Hepatitis Hotline . . . . . . . . . . . . . . . . . . . . . . . . . . . . . . . . . . . . . . . . . . . . . . . . . . 1-800-223-0179

National Clinicians' Post-Exposure Prophylaxis Hotline . . . . . . . . . . . . . . . . . . . . 1-888-448-4911

National Sexually Transmitted Disease Hotline . . . . . . . . . . . . . . . . . . . . . . . . . . . 1-800-227-8922

The publication, *The Health Hotlines*, which may be ordered from the National Library of Medicine, Office of Public Information, lists over 300 national hotlines. A free copy may be ordered by calling 800-272-4787.

## OTHER PUBLICATIONS BY THE NATIONAL ACUPUNCTURE FOUNDATION

### Acupuncture & Oriental Medicine State Laws and Regulations, 2005 Edition

Details the laws in all of the states in the United States. Includes detailed information on eligibility and examination requirements, scope of practice, fees, etc. for those states that have legislation.
ISBN 0-9670262-9-6

### Clean Needle Technique Manual, 5th Edition

The 5th edition of this standard publication in safe handling of acupuncture needles and equipment represents a comprehensive revision of previous material and an increase of nearly 20 pages of new material. It is the manual recommended by the Council of Colleges of Acupuncture and Oriental Medicine for study for the Clean Needle Technique Exam which is part of the national certification process for acupuncture and Oriental medicine professionals.
ISBN 0-9670262-6-1 (English language)
ISBN 0-9670262-7-X (Chinese language)
ISBN 0-9670262-8-8 (Korean language)

### Legal Issues in Integrative Medicine, by Michael H. Cohen

Provides basic guidance for those seeking to understand the legal context in which they offer integrative healthcare services to patients.
ISBN 0-9762537-0-4

Find these books and more information about the NAF on our web site:
**www.nationalacupuncturefoundation.org**

# Bibliography

"APIC Guidelines for Handwashing and Hand Antisepsis in Health-Care Settings", *American Journal of Infection Control* 23:251-269 (1995)

"APIC Guideline for Selection and Use of Disinfectants," *American Journal of Infection Control* 24, No. 4 (August 1996), pp. 313-342.

Beltrami, EM, Williams IT, Shapiro, CN and Chamberland, ME, "Risk and Management of Blood-Borne Infections in Health Care Workers," *Clinical Microbiology Reviews* 13, No. 3 (July 2000, pp. 385-407).

Boyce, JM, et al., Proceedings of the 9th Annual Society for Healthcare Epidemiology of America Meeting, April 18-20, 1999, San Francisco, CA.

CDCP, "Infection Control In Dentistry: Bloodborne Disease Transmission", *Promotion:* Division of Oral Health, July 3, 2000

Centers for Disease Control and Prevention, Immunization of Health-Care workers: Recommendations of the Advisory Committee on Immunization Practices (ACIP)

29 *CFR* 1910.1030 (d)(3)(ix).

CFR, 56, No. 235 (December 6, 1991), 64010 - 12

CFR 56, No. 235 (December 1991) 64116 -17

*Federal Register* (Washington, D.C.: U.S. Dept. of Labor, 52 no. 155, Aug. 12, 1987), 30082-30108, 21 *CFR* Part 872, Medical Devices: Dental Devices Classification; Final Rule and Withdrawal of Proposed Rule.

Gayle, HD and Hill, GL, "Global Impact of Human Immunodeficiency Virus and AIDS," *Clinical Microbiology Reviews* 14, No. 2 (April 2001) p. 327

Iippolito, et. al., "The Risk of Occupational Human Immunodeficiency Virus Infection in Health Care Workers," *Arch Intern Med* 153 (1993), 1456

Issues in Healthcare Settings "Sterilization or Disinfection of Medical Devices: General Principles", *Division of Healthcare Quality Promotion,* CDC 6/6/00

Lao, Li Xing, "Safety Issues in Acupuncture," *Journal of Alternative Medicine,* 2. No. 1 (Spring 1996)

MMWR 6/29/01 50 (RR11);1-42

Miller, Chris, "Heat Sterilization Assures Microbe-Free Instruments," *Dentist* (November-December, 1987), 26

National Acupuncture Foundation, *Safety Record of Acupuncture* (2002)

Potter, Fundamentals of Nursing (5th edition, 2001)

OSHA "Safe Needle Devices: Protecting Health Care Workers", October 1997.

Rodts, Mary and Benson, Daniel, "HIV Precautions for Prevention in the Workplace," *Orthopaedic Nursing* 11 No. 5 (September/October, 1992), 52-3.

Saulter, Gilbert J., Regional Administrator, OSHA Administration, Dallas, Texas, letter, November 25, 1994.

Stroffolini T, Lorenzoni U, Menniti-Ippolito F, Infantolino D, Chiaramonte M, Hepatitis C virus infection in spouses: sexual transmission or common exposure to the same risk factors? *Am J Gastroenterol.* 2001 Nov; 96(96):3051-3

The Hospital Infection Control Practices Advisory Committee (HICPAC), MMR 1997; 46 (No. RR18).

The Bloodborne Pathogens Standard, A Pragmatic Approach, O'Neal, Jon T., M.D., M.P.H. and Reinhold, Van Nostrand, New York, page 9, 1996.

Weinstein, Robert A., "Controlling Antimicrobial Resistance in Hospitals: Infection Control and Use of Antibiotics", Emerging Infectious Diseases, Vol. 7, No.2, Mar-Apr 2001.

"Updated U.S. Public Health Service Guidelines for the Management of Occupational Exposures to HBV, HCV and HIV and Recommendations for Postexposure Prophylaxis", MMWR, 6/29/01/50(RR/1); pp. 1-42.

Yee LJ, Weiss HL, Langer RG, Hererra J, Kaslow RA, Leeuwen DJ, "Risk factors for acquisition of hepatitis C virus infection: a case series and potential implications for disease surveillance," *BMC Infect Dis* 2001; 1:8

# Index

Alcohol . . . . . . . . . . . . . . . . . . . . . . . . . . . . . . . 24
Accidents . . . . . . . . . . . . . . . . . . . . . . . . . . . . . 53
Acupuncture needles
    Choosing, inspecting packaging . . . . . . . . . . . . . 18
    Disposable needles recommended . . . . . . . . . . . 18
    Disposal . . . . . . . . . . . . . . . . . . . . . . . 29, 30
    For electroacupuncture . . . . . . . . . . . . . . . . . 58
    Insertion . . . . . . . . . . . . . . . . . . . . 24, 25, 28
    Plum-blossom needles . . . . . . . . . . . . . . . . . 19
    Reusable needles . . . . . . . . . . . . . . . . . . . . 18
    Sterilization . . . . . . . . . . . . . . . . . . . . . . . 37
Autoclave . . . . . . . . . . . . . . . . . . . . . . . . . . . . 39
    Ensuring proper functioning . . . . . . . . . . . . . 45
    Load logs . . . . . . . . . . . . . . . . . . . . . . . . . 44
    Records . . . . . . . . . . . . . . . . . . . . . . . . . . 45
Autogenous infections . . . . . . . . . . . . . . . . . . . . . 2
Biohazardous waste . . . . . . . . . . . . . . . . . . . . . 30
Biological indicators . . . . . . . . . . . . . . . . . . . . . 44
Bleeding
    During cupping . . . . . . . . . . . . . . . . . . . . . . 29
    Techniques . . . . . . . . . . . . . . . . . . . . . . . . 59
Blood
    Contact . . . . . . . . . . . . . . . . . . . . . . . . . . 28
    Cleaning spill . . . . . . . . . . . . . . . . . . . . . . . 30
Broken Needle . . . . . . . . . . . . . . . . . . . . . . . . . 56
CNT Protocols . . . . . . . . . . . . . . . . . . . . . . . . . 13
    Basic principles . . . . . . . . . . . . . . . . . . . . . . 13
    Categories . . . . . . . . . . . . . . . . . . . . . . . . . 14
    Definitions . . . . . . . . . . . . . . . . . . . . . . . . 15
    Establishing a clean work area . . . . . . . . . . . . 20
Cross-Infections . . . . . . . . . . . . . . . . . . . . . . . . . 2
Cupping
    Cleaning equipment . . . . . . . . . . . . . . . . 19, 30
    Devices . . . . . . . . . . . . . . . . . . . . . . . . . . . 19
Disinfectants
    Classification and types . . . . . . . . . . . . . . . . 39
    Definition . . . . . . . . . . . . . . . . . . . . . . . . . 15
    Labeling . . . . . . . . . . . . . . . . . . . . . . . . . . 21
    Use in preliminary sterilization . . . . . . . . . . . 41
    Use on office surfaces . . . . . . . . . . . . . . . . . 20
Electrical stimulation . . . . . . . . . . . . . . . . . . . . . 58
Equipment . . . . . . . . . . . . . . . . . . . . . . . . . . . 18
Fainting . . . . . . . . . . . . . . . . . . . . . . . . . . . . . 55
Guide tubes . . . . . . . . . . . . . . . . . . . . . . . . 19, 25
Gloves . . . . . . . . . . . . . . . . . . . . . . . . 26, 52, 59
Handwashing . . . . . . . . . . . . . . . . . . . . . . . . . 21
    Alternatives to soap and water . . . . . . . . . . . . 23
    Immunocompromised patients . . . . . . . . . . . . 22
Hepatitis . . . . . . . . . . . . . . . . . . . . . . . . . . . . . . 3
    Chronic carriers . . . . . . . . . . . . . . . . . . . . . . 8
    Hepatitis A . . . . . . . . . . . . . . . . . . . . . . . . . 3
    Hepatitis B . . . . . . . . . . . . . . . . . . . . . . . . . 4

Hepatitis C . . . . . . . . . . . . . . . . . . . . . . . . . . . . 7
Hepatitis D . . . . . . . . . . . . . . . . . . . . . . . . . . . . 7
Hepatitis E . . . . . . . . . . . . . . . . . . . . . . . . . . . . 8
High-risk patients . . . . . . . . . . . . . . . . . . . . . . . 58
HIV . . . . . . . . . . . . . . . . . . . . . . . . . . . . . . . . . 9
    Infection process . . . . . . . . . . . . . . . . . . . . . 11
    Testing . . . . . . . . . . . . . . . . . . . . . . . . . . . 11
    Transmission . . . . . . . . . . . . . . . . . . . . . . . . 9
    Treatment . . . . . . . . . . . . . . . . . . . . . . . . . 12
Immune response . . . . . . . . . . . . . . . . . . . . . . . . 1
Informed consent . . . . . . . . . . . . . . . . . . . . . . . 48
Moxibustion . . . . . . . . . . . . . . . . . . . . . . . . . . 59
Needle insertion
    Depth . . . . . . . . . . . . . . . . . . . . . . . . . . . 28
    Injury to internal organs . . . . . . . . . . . . . . . . 57
    Pain or trauma after insertion . . . . . . . . . . . . 55
    Palpating the point . . . . . . . . . . . . . . . . . . . 24
    Positioning the patient . . . . . . . . . . . . . . . . . 21
    Preparing the site . . . . . . . . . . . . . . . . . . . . 24
Needlestick
    Accidental . . . . . . . . . . . . . . . . . . . . . . . . . 54
    Use of gloves . . . . . . . . . . . . . . . . . . . . . . . 26
OSHA exposure control plan . . . . . . . . . . . . . . . . 50
Patient confidentiality . . . . . . . . . . . . . . . . . . . . 49
Patient records . . . . . . . . . . . . . . . . . . . . . . . . 48
Practitioner recommendations . . . . . . . . . . . . . . . 16
    Clothing . . . . . . . . . . . . . . . . . . . . . . . . . . 16
    Hand care . . . . . . . . . . . . . . . . . . . . . . . . . 16
    If HIV or HBV positive . . . . . . . . . . . . . . . . . 16
    Personal health . . . . . . . . . . . . . . . . . . . . . . 16
    Testing for TB, HBV, HCV and HIV . . . . . . . . . 16
    Yearly physical . . . . . . . . . . . . . . . . . . . . . . 16
Public health settings . . . . . . . . . . . . . . . . . . . . 31
Spill
    Blood or body fluid . . . . . . . . . . . . . . . . . . . 30
    Used needles . . . . . . . . . . . . . . . . . . . . . . . 29
Sharps container . . . . . . . . . . . . . . . . . . . . . . . 29
Sterilization . . . . . . . . . . . . . . . . . . . . . . . . . . 37
    Autoclave . . . . . . . . . . . . . . . . . . . . . . . . . 38
    Chemical disinfectants . . . . . . . . . . . . . . . . . 39
    Double sterilization procedure . . . . . . . . . . . . 41
    Dry heat . . . . . . . . . . . . . . . . . . . . . . . . . . 39
    Monitoring . . . . . . . . . . . . . . . . . . . . . . . . 43
    Summary . . . . . . . . . . . . . . . . . . . . . . . . . 46
Stuck needle . . . . . . . . . . . . . . . . . . . . . . . . . . 56
Travel Kit . . . . . . . . . . . . . . . . . . . . . . . . . . . . 34
Universal Precautions (summary) . . . . . . . . . . . . . 51
Vaccination
    HAV . . . . . . . . . . . . . . . . . . . . . . . . . . . . . 3
    HBV . . . . . . . . . . . . . . . . . . . . . . . . . . . . . 5

ISBN 0-9670262-6-1

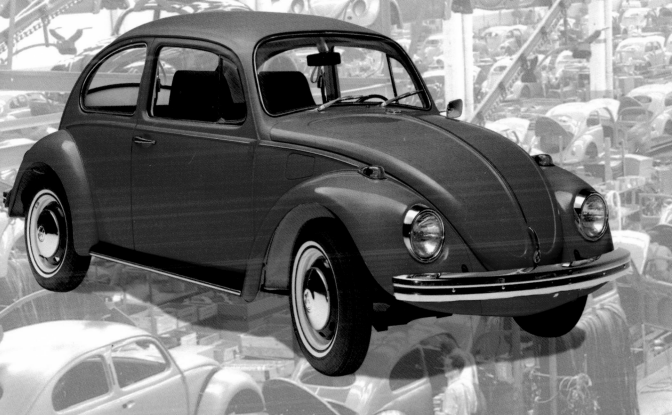

# The VW BEETLE

## A Production History of the World's Most Famous Car, 1936–1967

**RYAN LEE PRICE**

ISBN 1-55788-421-8

EAN